ANOREXIA

ANOREXIA

Stacy Beller Stryer

Biographies of Disease
Julie K. Silver, M.D., Series Editor

GREENWOOD PRESS
An Imprint of ABC-CLIO, LLC

A B C 🔖 C L I O

Santa Barbara, California • Denver, Colorado • Oxford, England

Library of Congress Cataloging-in-Publication Data

Stryer, Stacy Beller.
    Anorexia / Stacy Beller Stryer.
        p. cm. — (Biographies of disease)
    Includes bibliographical references and index.
    ISBN 0-313-35975-X (hard copy : alk. paper) — ISBN 0-313-35976-8 (ebook)
1. Anorexia nervosa—Popular works. I. Title.
    RC552.A5S87 2009
    616.85'262—dc22   2009024108

13 12 11 10 9   1 2 3 4 5

This book is also available on the World Wide Web as an eBook.
Visit www.abc-clio.com for details.

ABC-CLIO, LLC
130 Cremona Drive, P.O. Box 1911
Santa Barbara, California 93116-1911

This book is printed on acid-free paper ∞

Manufactured in the United States of America

Copyright Acknowledgments

The author wishes to thank Arianne Waschler for her advice and autobiographical
contribution provided throughout the book.

To Rachael and Becca,
Whose love and encouragement
Inspire me beyond words

In memory of Dan,
My eternal cheerleader

Contents

Series Foreword

Every disease has a story to tell: about how it started long ago and began to disable or even take the lives of its innocent victims, about the way it hurts us, and about how we are trying to stop it. In this Biographies of Disease series, the authors tell the stories of the diseases that we have come to know and dread.

The stories of these diseases have all of the components that make for great literature. There is incredible drama played out in real-life scenes from the past, present, and future. You'll read about how men and women of science stumbled trying to save the lives of those they aimed to protect. Turn the pages and you'll also learn about the amazing success of those who fought for health and won, often saving thousands of lives in the process.

If you don't want to be a health professional or research scientist now, when you finish this book you may think differently. The men and women in this book are heroes who often risked their own lives to save or improve ours. This is the biography of a disease, but it is also the story of real people who made incredible sacrifices to stop it in its tracks.

Julie K. Silver, M.D.
Assistant Professor, Harvard Medical School
Department of Physical Medicine and Rehabilitation

Preface

A norexia nervosa is a mental illness which has been identified for over a century, but its incidence has increased dramatically only in the past 40 to 50 years. Although it was once rare and unfamiliar within the general population, it is now easily recognized by most people. *Anorexia* is written to examine the history of self-starvation from ancient times through present day, and the potential impact of Western culture, society, and economy on the desire to be thin. The text also discusses prominent theories of why self-starvation occurs and how best to treat it. The book is written in a chronological and easy-to-follow manner, allowing the reader to follow the progression of self-starvation through time and the birth of a new mental illness.

Furthermore, it provides the opportunity to understand firsthand what it is like to have this illness. Interspersed throughout the chapters are quotes and comments by Arianne Waschler, a third-year college student who developed anorexia during her junior year of high school. Although she had an extremely difficult two years, "Ari" received treatment early and was doing well enough to graduate high school on time and begin college the following fall. *Anorexia* is to be used by students and others who want to have a thorough and complete understanding of this illness, both from a historical and present-day perspective.

ACKNOWLEDGMENTS

I wish to thank Arianne Waschler for her advice and the autobiographical contributions she provided throughout the book.

I would like to thank Julie K. Silver for providing me with the opportunity to write this book, and Kevin Downing for patiently answering my numerous questions and guiding me through this endeavor. I also want to thank my esteemed colleagues, who generously gave their time to review the book, including Heather Prescott, Bronwen Williams, and Vivian Mehan. In addition, I am grateful to my family and friends who spent numerous hours reviewing my manuscript and providing suggestions, including Debbie Auerbach Deutsch, Clotilde Puertolas, Nancy Beller-Simms, David Gillette, Joan Beller, William Beller, Lubert Stryer, and Andrea Stenn Stryer. I would particularly like to thank my niece, Ari. Not only did she spend hours talking to me about her journey with anorexia, but she also had the courage and desire to help others by telling her story, which is still so fresh in her mind.

Introduction

P eople, particularly women, have been starving themselves since the Biblical period and, some say, even longer. Throughout the centuries, those
who severely limit their food intake have given many different explanations, including an attempt to purify the soul or to demonstrate devotion to
God, a belief that food is not necessary to sustain life, and a fear of becoming
fat. The reasons people have given during a particular time period appear to
have changed as the social, cultural, and economic environments have evolved.

The idea that self-starvation may actually be abnormal or an illness unique
from others was not fully developed until the late 1800s when an English physician, William Gull, and a French physician, Charles Laségue, simultaneously
described several patients who appeared physically healthy yet were refusing to
eat. Gull coined the name "anorexia nervosa," which, although the term does
not correctly define the illness, is still used today. The term *anorexia* means *loss
of appetite*, and *nervosa* means *nervous*, yet those who are affected do not lose
their appetite but willingly refuse to eat and, although they have many anxieties surrounding food, their illness is not due to nerves or being nervous. For
several years after Gull's and Laségue's initial descriptions, only limited interest was paid to this group of patients. Eventually, psychiatrists, endocrinolo-
gists, and other physicians began to present a variety of theories and possible

treatments for anorexia nervosa. Nevertheless, there was no clear cut definition of the illness until 1980, when criteria needed to make the diagnosis of anorexia were first published in the major reference book used by mental health professionals in the United States.

Major changes which occurred in Western society throughout the twentieth century, especially for women, most likely contributed to the dramatic rise in anorexia nervosa. Socially, there was the birth and growth of feminism. Women began to demand opportunities for higher education and a place in the workforce. Culturally, women shed their formal individually designed outfits and began to purchase clothes which were tighter, exposed more of their bodies, and were produced in factories, and came in standard sizes. Mass media began to advertise the benefits of looking good for others, not just on the inside, but also on the outside, and publishers began to introduce dieting books. By the 1960s, the media had significantly shifted their focus to the superficial qualities of women, and the entertainment industry routinely chose ultra-thin actresses and models, such as Twiggy, to represent the perfect modern woman.

The incidence of anorexia nervosa has significantly increased over the past few decades and, consequently, there has been an increase in research on the possible causes and treatments of anorexia. Theories have evolved over the past century from considering those affected to be hysterical; to claiming they have an endocrine abnormality; to considering them victims of a combination of factors, including heredity, family dynamics, and biochemical abnormalities. Likewise, treatment recommendations have also changed with time from warm bed rest and force feeding, to years of psychoanalysis, to multiple-therapy treatments involving families, nutritionists, and group therapists. Researchers are continuing to search for the possible causes of and best treatment for anorexia nervosa, in addition to ways to prevent children from developing it. Since multiple studies are being conducted on so many different aspects of anorexia, the hope is that better methods to prevent, diagnose, and treat anorexia are just around the corner.

1

The History of Self-Starvation

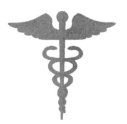

My initials are AN. For a time period, they represented anorexia nervosa, but that illness no longer defines me. My name is Arianne Nicole, and I will forever be connected to anorexia nervosa, even though I have fully recovered.

—Ari

Anorexia nervosa is one of the most common psychiatric diagnoses in young women today. Approximately 0.6% to 1% of female adolescents in the United States suffer from anorexia nervosa. This translates to 7 million women.

90% to 95% of those who have anorexia nervosa are women.

About 1 million men suffer from anorexia nervosa.

86% of those affected developed their illness before age 20, and 10% reported onset at age 10 years or younger.

Without treatment or with prolonged illness, up to 20% of people who suffer from anorexia will die as a result of their disease, making it the mental illness with the highest risk of mortality

(Anorexia Nervosa and Associated Eating Disorders n.d.)

norexia nervosa is a term familiar to all of us. Whether we are watching gymnasts perform their aerial maneuvers, ballerinas dance on Pointe in the holiday classic "The Nutcracker," or models gracefully walk down a runway, we are acutely aware of their size and shape. At times we notice a performer who appears to be painfully thin and we automatically assume, almost too flippantly, that she must have anorexia nervosa (also called "anorexia"). Yet 40 years ago chances are that thoughts about anorexia, or any other eating disorder, would not have crossed anybody's mind because most people had never heard of it. Although anorexia has been recognized since the late 1800s, it wasn't until the 1970s that physicians and the general population really became aware of this mental illness. Unfortunately, the sudden increase in awareness is most likely due to a rapid rise in the incidence of anorexia which began in the mid-1960s.

As greater numbers of anorexics were being recognized, more information became available to the public. By the early 1970s, articles about anorexia were found in magazines and newspapers, books, and even on television. According to Joan Jacobs Brumberg, author of "Fasting Girls," an article in the *Science Digest* in the early 1970s referred to anorexia as a "strange new disease" where teen girls had a morbid fear of eating. Other magazines, such as *People*, *Mademoiselle*, and *Seventeen* began to publish articles about anorexia and its extreme effects. Newspapers such as the *New York Times* published specific information for the first time about the disease, such as the mortality rate (reported numbers varied from 5% to 50%) and various treatments available for anorexia (Brumberg 1997). In 1973 and again in 1978, Hilde Bruch, a pediatrician and psychoanalyst who was one of the world's leading experts on eating disorders, published two significant books that further increased our understanding and knowledge regarding anorexia. The first, *Eating Disorders: Obesity, Anorexia Nervosa and the Person Within*, was written primarily for professionals (Bruch 1973), whereas the second, *The Golden Cage: The Enigma of Anorexia Nervosa*, was written for the lay person (Bruch 1978). A year later, a fictional character named Kessa was portrayed as an anorexic in a fictional book, *The Best Little Girl in the World*, which was made into a TV movie (Levenkron 1978). Soon portrayals of anorexia were everywhere, including TV comedies such as "Saturday Night Live" where, in 1984, they told several jokes about anorexia and showed what a cookbook for anorexics might look like.

THE SIGNIFICANCE OF SELF-STARVATION

Self-starvation is not a new phenomenon. People have willingly starved themselves since the Biblical period, or even longer. Even so, it was not until the 1600s that Dr. Richard Morton provided us with the first descriptions of what might be considered modern-day anorexia. It took another 200 years before two prominent physicians, Drs. William Gull and Charles Laségue, recognized and described anorexia as a condition unique from others that were also associated with emaciation and weight loss. Does this mean that anorexia nervosa didn't exist before the 1800s? Is it a new disease? These are not easy questions to answer, and historians have argued both sides of the issue (Vandereycken and van Deth 1994). Before proceeding, anorexia nervosa needs to be defined. Individuals with anorexia must weigh 85% or less than that which is expected for their height, gender, and age. They also need to have an intense fear of gaining weight and becoming fat. In addition, they must either deny that their weight is a problem, directly associate their body weight and shape with their self-worth, or think that they are overweight when, in reality, they are too thin. Finally, menstruating females must have amenorrhea (the lack of periods) for at least three cycles (American Psychiatric Association 2000).

THE DEBATE SURROUNDING ANOREXIA NERVOSA

Most present-day historians and physicians agree that the patients described by Gull and Laségue in the 1870s had anorexia nervosa. These prominent physicians wrote about their patients in detail, including the significant weight loss, physical and mental changes, and fear of gaining weight, all without evidence of being afflicted with any specific medical illness. Their descriptions are similar to those given today to illustrate individuals with anorexia. Some historians, such as Tilmann Habermas, Ron van Deth, and Walter Vandereycken, believe that anorexia nervosa is, by definition, a modern phenomenon and did not exist before the mid-1800s because there is no documentation before this period that individuals starved themselves because they feared becoming fat. These historians surmise that if a weight concern wasn't mentioned by a physician, it should be taken as evidence that the physician was not worried about it and not that the physician was oblivious to weight issues. Habermas uses the example of a physician, Dr. Worthington, who, in 1875, documented a case regarding a patient who fasted excessively to control her weight. Since Worthington was aware of such issues, other physicians must have been aware of them also and, therefore, would have documented weight problems if they existed. Habermas also argues that both Drs. Gull and Laségue documented cases of patients who starved themselves to control their weight or because they were afraid of gaining weight. Furthermore, the fact that both physicians documented more cases toward the end of the century could signify an increase in the incidence of weight fears as the century progressed (Habermas 2005). Habermas, van Deck and Vandereycken make one more point in that one can't assume what is not written in historical records; through historical research they were unable to locate any documentation of an association between self-starvation and the fear of gaining weight before the mid-1800s.

Other historians, including Pamela Keel, Kelly Klump, and Joseph Silverman, disagree and hypothesize that there may have been sociocultural reasons physicians didn't document or identify anorexia prior to the 1870s but, nevertheless, that it still may have existed (Keel and Klump 2003). For example, women may have been afraid to gain weight or felt that they were fat although they were actually extremely thin. Since they weren't as open about their thoughts or feelings as they are today, they may not have told anybody. Keel and Klump also argue that weight loss and signs of self-starvation may have been ignored by others or attributed to conditions which were common during that time period, such as hysteria or nervousness during the 19th century (Gordon 2000).

In addition to proposing that there may have been sociocultural reasons for not identifying anorexics in previous centuries, Keel and Klump also believe that fear of gaining weight is a culturally-bound belief for a more important underlying problem. Therefore, they propose that changing the definition to accommodate cultural differences could lead to the diagnosis of anorexia nervosa in people earlier than the nineteenth century. Although society currently associates self-starvation with the desire to be thin, in previous centuries there may have been other culturally relevant reasons. Dr. Joseph Silverman proposed that the criteria be changed to include a dramatic weight loss evident to others; symptoms of prolonged starvation, such as hypothermia, constipation, bradycardia (low heart rate), and lanugo (fine hair that grows on body of people who are starving); the lack of a known medical or psychiatric illness; significant hyperactivity; and the denial that weight loss is a problem, such as by refusing to seek help (Silverman 1983).

Also, information available today may not have existed previously; therefore, those living in prior eras may have been naïve about what it means to be underweight or overweight. For example, they didn't have the instruments with which to measure themselves or to compare themselves to others because scales and mirrors were not a part of many households until the late 1800s. In addition, they had no idea what "normal weight" was. Standard charts that indicated what weight was normal or appropriate for a given height and gender were not published until the turn of the century. Keel and Klump propose that it is the idea that someone intentionally starves themselves without the ability to stop which is important, rather than the actual fear of gaining weight or the acknowledgment that fasting and weight loss are causing problems. They believe there are many similarities between people who starved themselves centuries ago and modern-day anorexics. They were often female and from the upper echelon of society. They were perfectionists, began their starvation at an early age, stopped menstruating, became hyperactive, had a decreased sexual drive, and developed strange eating habits. Others often tried to persuade those who were starving themselves to stop, but they were unsuccessful.

Independent of the reason, it is evident that self-starvation has occurred for centuries. The reasons people give for voluntarily starving themselves change over time based on the cultural environment. It is important to remember that, just as society evolves over time, so do the reasons people give for starving themselves. Thus, at any point in time, most people will provide one reason for refusing food while a few will state reasons heard years earlier and reasons which will be heard more frequently in the future. Common historical themes and explanations for self-starvation include, but are not limited to:

- Religious cleansing of sins
- Preparation for a special religious event
- Cure for illness
- Religious asceticism
- Demonic possession
- Being a witch
- Miracles
- Trying to gain attention and/or make money
- Having hysteria, a gastric illness, or a nervous disease
- Female gender

SELF-STARVATION EXISTED IN THE BIBLICAL PERIOD AND BEYOND

According to the Old Testament, fasting was common during the Biblical period and was often used as a means of self-humiliation and self-castigation; or a way to "cleanse oneself from previous sins." It was also performed after the death of an important political or religious figure, as part of the preparation for an important religious experience, to purify oneself, and to prove devotion to God. Many religious figures reportedly fasted to receive dreams, visions, and revelations from higher powers. A nonreligious purpose for fasting was to treat various ailments and physical conditions (Vandereycken and van Deth 1994). There are many examples of fasting for these purposes. More than 2,500 years ago, Jews fasted after Gedaliah ben Ahikam, the Governor of Judah, was assassinated. Religious figures, including Moses and Jesus, fasted for 40 days to become in a trance-like state so they could receive visions. Moses fasted before he went to Mt. Sinai to receive the Ten Commandments, and Jesus fasted in the desert to be tested and tempted by Satan. From the first century through the fourth century, men who belonged to various cults fasted and lived as hermits because they wanted to deny themselves any physical or material comforts. During the late fourth century, a 20-year old woman died from severe malnutrition secondary to fasting. She was a follower of St. Jerome, a priest and spiritual leader of a group of wealthy Roman women. He believed in abstinence, prayer, and fasting, and encouraged his followers to do the same to live a more Christian life. The death of his follower may be the first time in history that death due to self-starvation has been recorded (Bemporad 1996). Several well-known Greco-Roman physicians, including Galen (131–201) and Alexander of Trallianus (525–605), recommended fasting to cure various medical conditions. Galen believed that "humors" were formed in the body and different foods could have an effect on the humors; their imbalance could cause disease. He recommended various treatments to restore their balance, including starvation and purging. The herbs he prescribed were emetics, laxatives, diuretics, and enemas. Galen's theories remained popular throughout the Middle Ages.

The incidence of self-starvation decreased during the early Middle Ages. Interestingly, the number of documented cases of fasting has varied throughout history, with greater numbers recorded during times of economic wealth and fewer numbers recorded during times of economic difficulty. For example, the early Middle Ages was a time of chaos, rampages, famine, death due to the plague, and breakdown of society. Cities were demolished and people feared for their lives and livelihood. According to the psychiatrist, Dr. Jules Bemporad, the number of people who starved themselves during this difficult period decreased dramatically. Bemporad discusses that one possibility is that historical records were not kept as well during the early Middle Ages as they had been previously. An alternative explanation, however, is that the decrease in the incidence of self-starvation was accurate and because it did not carry much significance during this era, there was no incentive to voluntarily starve oneself. After all, it is difficult to make a personal or political statement, or to draw attention to oneself as being unique by consciously refusing food when much of society is involuntarily starving. The few documented stories of self-starvation during this period included women who were reportedly possessed by the devil and one of a princess who lived between 700 and 900 A.D. While she was single, she made a vow of virginity to God. After she made her promise, her father told her she was to be married. Because of her desire to remain loyal to God, she refused to eat and "grew hair all over her body" (Bemporad 1996). Her father had her crucified, and years later she became Saint Liberata. A modern day example of decreased self-starvation during difficult times occurred in Italy during World War II. A well-known Italian psychiatrist, Dr. Mara Selvini Palazzoli, wrote that anorexia nervosa was almost nonexistent during the war, a time of significant food restrictions. After the war was over and Italians began to do better financially, anorexia resurfaced. Dr. Selvini Palazzoli surmised that the disappearance of anorexia was due to the poor economy.

During the Middle Ages, religious, sociocultural and economic changes arose throughout Europe, which set the stage for the next type of individual who practiced self-starvation. Interestingly, most cases from this point until modern times described women from more Western societies, such as England, France, and the United States. Religion took center stage for several centuries. Christianity had already become the major religion of the Roman Empire during the third century, and it continued to spread throughout parts of Africa, Asia, and all of Europe. By 800, Western Europe was ruled by Christian Kings, and the Pope became not only a spiritual leader, but also an important political leader throughout Christian society. According to the Church, people by nature were sinners and were dependent on God's favor. To receive his approval, they were required to take part in sacraments, one of the most important being the Eucharist. During this sacrament, eating a special piece of bread was taken as evidence of receiving Jesus' invisible presence, as his body was in the bread. These sacraments continue in the Catholic Church today, and those who partake in it are expected to fast and confess their sins prior to receiving communion.

By the tenth and eleventh centuries, many aspects of life began to improve for Europeans, which led to the emergence of a middle class. As the economy improved through business and trade, education and the arts also began to thrive. Along with all of these changes came a significant increase in self-starvation which centered on religious pursuits. Around 1200, devout Christians began to fast for ascetic reasons. Asceticism, which is a type of self-denial performed to try to attain spiritual perfection, mainly occurred among relatively young religious females who claimed to eat little or nothing for years. Some reportedly subsisted solely on the Eucharist, or the presence of Jesus. Their reasons for fasting coincided with the Catholic Church's ideals, as the Church not only supported, but promoted fasting. It equated hunger with holiness and actually required many fasts throughout the year to prove religious devotion. When stories spread of the girls who were able to survive on so little food for months to years, it was considered a miracle. Even though some of these women admitted that they were ill and were physically unable to eat, their self-starvation was still considered a wonder. The Catholic Church named many women who successfully starved themselves, such as St. Wilge-fortis and St. Margaret, as saints. Through research, historian Rudolph Bell discovered 261 cases of women who fasted for ascetic purposes, most occurring through 1200 and 1600 in Southern Europe. He named these women "Holy Anorexics" (Bell 1985).

One well-known story of such a holy anorexic was Catherine of Siena (1347–1380) (Figure 1.1). As a teenager, Catherine refused to marry but instead wanted to become a nun. However, before she left home, her older sister died.

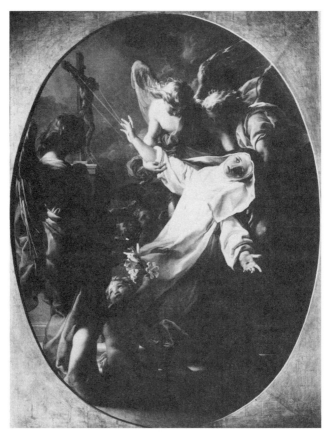

Figure 1.1. Catherine of Siena. Saint Catherine of Siena, 1347–1380, was one of many women who practiced self-starvation and devoted their lives to the Church. She died from strokes and malnutrition secondary to starvation. Such women were called "holy maidens." [Photo courtesy of Art Resource]

Catherine decided to fast, and she rarely ate anything but a handful of herbs each day. When she was forced to eat, she shoved twigs down her throat to bring up the food. Apparently, she developed limitless amounts of energy despite the fact that the amount of sleep she required decreased to one to two hours a night. Similar symptoms are seen in anorexics today. Although she spent the first few years after her sister's death as a hermit, she eventually left her home and became a nun. She died at age 33 from malnutrition and a series of strokes due to starvation. Other well-known stories from this time period include those of Alpais of Cudot, Mary of Oignes, and Beatrice of Nazareth. Reportedly, Alpais of Cudot ate nothing but the Eucharist from 1170–1211. Mary of Oignes and Beatrice of Nazareth, who lived during the thirteenth century, vomited from the smell of meat, and their throats are said to have swelled shut in the presence of food (Brumberg 2000). Despite their self-starvation, they were often very active physically and appeared to be unbothered by their lack of sustenance.

RELIGIOUS REFORMATION IMPACTS SELF-STARVATION

The end of the Middle Ages coincided with growing opposition to the Catholic Church and the Protestant Reformation during the 1500s. Changes occurred with regard to religious beliefs and worship practices, including those of ascetic fasting. Whereas fasting was encouraged to show devotion to God and Jesus before the Reformation, it became openly discouraged after. In addition, many fewer holy anorexics became saints, and the Protestant Church refuted the idea that religious followers needed to starve or deny themselves sustenance to prove self devotion to God. As this idea gained acceptance, the number of girls who reportedly starved for ascetic reasons decreased while the number who refused sustenance for other reasons was on the rise.

During the fifteenth and sixteenth centuries, many individuals, mostly women, who fasted were considered bewitched or possessed by demons. Although this theory existed prior to the fifteenth century, its popularity rose during this epoch. Even holy anorexics, including Catherine of Siena and Alpais of Cudot, were aware that individuals who fasted were being accused of these sins. They tried to eat just enough so that they would not be accused of such an evil, and also to assure themselves that they were not being tricked by the devil (Vandereycken and van Deth 1994). While Catherine and Alpais were successful at proving their holiness, others were not and some were eventually charged with witchcraft.

Many cases of possession or bewitchment occur in the literature during this time period. For example, Jane Stretton was thought to be possessed by the devil. Jane came from a rather religious family. Sometime around the end of the 1660s, her father lost a prized Bible and, on trying to find out who had taken it, he questioned a neighbor who said that he knew who had it. Jane's father thought that this man must have been the devil or a witch because he knew who took the Bible. One month later Jane began to have "raging fits," right around the time that the neighbor's wife gave her a pin for no known reason. Six months later Jane stopped eating and no longer produced any urine or stool. Because of her fragile state, she was watched continuously, during which time several observers saw flames and pins coming from her mouth. Jane's family and community concluded that she was possessed by their neighbors, both the devil and a witch. Eventually Jane's spell was broken, although she never ate solid foods again (Linton 1883).

NEW IDEAS ABOUT SELF-STARVATION DEVELOP

Around the sixteenth and seventeenth centuries the bewitchment theory began to lose popularity, although it still remained a cause for self-starvation in some individuals. The next theory applied to individuals who starved themselves for no known reason was simply that it was due to a miracle, so these people were referred to as "miraculous maidens." This group differed from the former in that they weren't religious and did not desire to show their holiness toward or devotion to religious figures. Because no cause could be found for their fasting, their miraculous stories spread from town to town and they became very well-known throughout the region. People often came from far away to see a person who survived on no food or liquids, and who produced no stool or urine. One story, which took place in 1585, exemplifies the attitudes of people during this era. Catharina Binder, who was by no means religious, reportedly survived without food for seven years. A local count, who was suspicious of her story, requested that a group of "respectable men" examine the situation and observe her. After two weeks, they concluded that she was telling the truth. As was often the case during these years, girls were examined by physicians or others who couldn't find a reason for their lack of eating, and their case was therefore considered a miracle (Vandereycken and van Deth 1994). Another famous case is that of 19-year old Martha Taylor of Derbyshire. Beginning in 1667, she reportedly ate nothing for over 13 months and only drank an occasional few drops of the syrup of stewed prunes or raisins, water, and sugar. Although she slept little and appeared emaciated "like a skeleton," she continued to be active. Once again, her story was considered a miracle by many. Others, however, began to wonder and question how someone could survive for such a long time without food (Silverman 1983). These cases are important because they document the time society, as a whole, began to question the cause of self-starvation, perhaps thinking about it more in medical terms.

Dr. Richard Morton

As scientists and the general population began to question whether the fasting girls could actually survive without eating for a prolonged period, they started to look for legitimate reasons behind their lack of eating. Dr. Richard Morton (1637–1698) is credited for being the first person to provide a detailed medical description of someone who may have had what we currently refer to as anorexia nervosa. His description is detailed in his *Treatise of Consumptions*, a book he wrote in 1689 (Malson 1998). Morton, a British physician, had a great reputation and was appointed as the physician in ordinary to King William III (Pearce 2004). In his *Treatise*, he discussed the need for accurate definitions of medical conditions. One of his examples was an illness called consumption, which is "a wasting disease of the muscular parts of the body." Morton discussed two types of consumption, original and symptomatical. The first type was due to an underlying medical illness, such as tuberculosis. The second type, also known as "nervous consumption" or "nervous atrophy," was not due to any known medical illness, nor did the patients have any symptoms of disease, such as a cough or fever. Morton said that the cause of symptomatical consumption, where individuals lose their appetite, is "purely from a Morbid Disposition of the Blood, or Animal Spirits, which reside in the System of the Nerves and Fibres, and is not the effect of any other preceding Disease" (Bhanji and Newton 1985). It is this type of consumption, the one where wasting occurred without any other evidence of disease, which people credit with possibly being modern day anorexia (Bhanji and Newton 1985).

Although Morton did not discuss how often he saw this type of consumption, he did speculate that it could be caused by "sadness and anxious cares," or alcohol. He recommended a specific treatment for these patients, including efforts to make them happy and carefree, provide tasty food, and expose the patient to fresh air. He also mentioned various homeopathic remedies, such as salts, specific wines, and various herbs. Morton observed that the earlier the problem was recognized, the easier it was to cure (Bhanji and Newton 1985).

Morton also discussed two cases in his *Treatise of Consumptions*. His descriptions of their weight loss and associated symptoms are similar to those observed in modern-day anorexics. The first case pertains to Mary Axe, who, in 1684, was 18 years old. She lost the ability to have periods because of "a multitude of Cares and Passions of her Mind, but without any Symptom of the Green-Sickness [a type of anemia] following upon it." According to

Morton, her flesh became "flaccid and loose" and her skin looked pale but, despite this, she continued to study and read books "day and night." Eventually she began to have fainting fits. When she was finally seen by Morton, she looked like "a Skeleton only clad with skin," and she had a very cold body but no other signs of a physical illness. Morton recommended several medicines and, although she appeared better after using some of them she decided to stop taking them and died three months later (Bhanji and Newton 1985).

Morton's second case was, interestingly, that of a 16-year-old boy. His account of his patient is that the boy "fell gradually into a total want of Appetite, occasioned by his studying too hard, and the Passions of his Mind" (Bhanji and Newton). Over the next two years he continued to lack an appetite but didn't exhibit any other signs of an illness. He was diagnosed as having a nervous consumption and tried a host of medications without any improvement. Morton advised him to stop studying, to relax in the country air, and to enjoy himself. The boy reportedly mostly recovered but was not totally without consumption (Pearce 2004).

Dr. Robert Whytt

Just as Morton was credited with being the first to give a detailed medical description of what may be anorexia nervosa, some consider Dr. Robert Whytt (1714–1766) to be the first to identify and record the biological changes that occur with severe fasting. In 1764, he published a paper in which he discussed "nervous atrophy," and then presented a case. He described a wasting of the body which was not due to a medical illness, nor was it specifically from the brain or nervous system but instead seemed to come from an "unnatural or morbid state of the nerves, of the stomach, and intestines." He observed that individuals who had this nervous atrophy also had a low spirit or melancholy which may have contributed to their malnutrition. The biological changes that Whytt recorded included not only the significant loss of flesh, but also the lack of sweats, the decreased core body temperature (hypothermia), and the low heart rate (bradycardia) which can accompany severe wasting (Silverman 1987a).

SELF-STARVATION IS EXAMINED IN FURTHER DETAIL

The way Morton and Whytt applied thought and deductive reasoning to those who were starving themselves exemplified the way society began to examine many aspects of life during the Renaissance Period and the Scientific Revolution, leading to new ideas and discoveries. Science became more important and many old thoughts and ideas were questioned, including teachings from the Catholic Church. Philosophers such as Francis Bacon and René Descartes combined scientific thought and philosophy and devised new ways of thinking about science, some of which we use today. Bacon thought truth came only after a complete evaluation of the evidence. This is called "the scientific method," where scientists try to prove a hypothesis by observation and/or experimentation. Descartes preached that truth must come from reason (Farah and Karls 2001). This new type of thinking was implemented in many ways, even with the miraculous maidens. Medical experts seriously began to question the authenticity of the maidens' starvation and the likelihood that they truly could survive for extended periods of time without any food. As more cases surfaced, many demanded that their stories be verified by knowledgeable, careful observers. Doctors speculated that these girls were actually fasting to gain notoriety or fame; or to make money.

As a result of careful, persistent questioning and observation, many imposters were revealed. One was Anne Moore of Tutbury, England (see Figure 1.2), who reportedly began to live without food in 1807. Attempts to observe and charge her as a fraud in 1808 failed and she became rather well-known as a "miraculous maiden." People came from all over England and paid to see her, so she made a fair bit of money. At first, her story appears similar to those of the miraculous maidens. However, the difference is that it didn't make sense medically, so physicians continued to question the authenticity of it. In 1813, a group of doctors demanded to observe her again, but this time they had to end their watch early because she became very sick. Her fraudulence and that of her family was soon discovered. She drank the liquid from the towels she used for washing because they contained gravy, milk, and strong arrowroot, as did the kisses she received from her mother (van Deth and Vandereycken 1993).

The story of Sarah Jacobs, the "Welsh Fasting Girl," is another example of a girl where, years earlier, people would simply have been satisfied with calling her a miraculous maiden but, due to persistent questioning and observation, was also found to be a fraud. In the 1860s, at 10 years of age, she was said to have stopped eating. A committee was formed and watched her for two weeks, but they could find no evidence of deceit. Initially, some people began to call her a miraculous faster. However, a physician named Dr. Robert Fowler believed that her fasting was not due to a miracle but to hysteria, a common diagnosis in the 1800s. Despite the reluctance of some, a second watch was organized where four nurses took turns observing her in her home. After just a few days she became very ill and, as her parents refused to feed her, she died before the end of her observation period (Bemporad 1996).

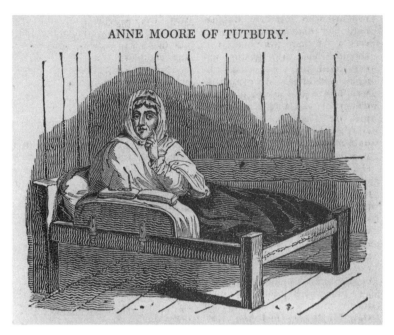

Figure 1.2. Anne Moore of Tutbury. She was a "miraculous maiden" who reportedly lived without food for no apparent reason. In 1813, after six years without food or water, she was carefully observed by a team of adults and was found to be a fraud. [Photo courtesy of Harvard College]

FASTING DURING THE VICTORIAN ERA

This new, original way of thinking which began during the Scientific Revolution continued through the Industrial Revolution in the mid-1800s. Innovations in agriculture and industry led to significant economic, social, and political changes. Materials for mass and rapid production were invented and factories were opened. Improved agricultural production led to safer foods, and better health caused a population explosion. All of these factors resulted in an increase in the size, power, and wealth of the middle class (Farah and Karls 2001).

By the Victorian Era, middle-class ideals about family roles began to change. Whereas previously every member of the family worked to keep food on the table, now middle-class men were usually the sole financial caretakers of the household while women focused on caring for their family and home. Individuality, independence, and self-fulfillment gained new, heightened importance, although these goals were mainly achievable by the men. There was new insight into individual feelings and the emotional aspects of relationships (Vandereycken and van Deth 1994). As middle-class mothers spent more time and energy preparing meals, food took on a new meaning, even being used as a form of affection and discipline. They worked hard at making their meals taste and look good. If a child didn't like a certain meal or refused to eat a particular food, a second helping may have been doled out and the child would have had to finish it before going to bed. If a child was being rewarded or punished for something, this often led to an extra helping or the denial of a certain meal or part of it, respectively. Whereas in previous periods in history, the upper classes differentiated themselves by offering greater quantities of food, during the Victorian era they began to offer smaller, tastier amounts. In fact, now women were supposed to be hungry and refuse sweets and other treats. Their refusal was a sign of self-control, intelligence, and high moral character, especially because certain foods and large quantities of food were related to increased sexual desire in women, which was frowned on.

Children also developed a more important and central role within the family. Parents paid more attention to them making various phases, such as adolescence, a more turbulent time for the family than it had been previously. Mothers, in particular, felt responsible for teaching their teens about hygiene, exercise, proper diets, and moral character. Emotions and feelings were openly expressed, and love gradually replaced authority as the center of family relations. Sometimes this caused an unhealthy dependence of one family member on another making one member feel suffocated, and other times, led to acts of manipulation. Food was an important symbol of love of a mother toward the rest of the family. Refusing to eat led to feelings of rejection and refusal of love. Yet it was one way a child could express discontent with a family situation (Brumberg 2000).

Although Morton and Whytt documented during the 1600s that self-starvation was due to a medical condition, it was not until the 1800s that several physicians began to notice that self-starvation was actually a symptom of a disease. Their discoveries came during a period which emphasized the importance of medical observation, description, and classification of diseases. The astute and detailed descriptions these physicians gave regarding adolescent girls with self-starvation are similar to those of modern-day anorexics. These physicians, who began to notice patients who were starving themselves, wanted to understand why some people, particularly seemingly healthy, privileged, young women, refused to eat. Not only did these girls starve themselves, but they also appeared sad and socially withdrawn. In addition, they developed amenorrhea, the loss of their monthly periods, and some had anemia—all without evidence of an organic illness.

WHAT PHYSICIANS THOUGHT ABOUT SELF-STARVATION IN THE 1800s

Although physicians from the early and mid-1800s tried to understand the cause of self-starvation in their patients, most used common afflictions from society to explain the cause. Many concluded that the cause was psychological and due to one of several mental illnesses which were commonly diagnosed during that time period. This included hysteria, nervous atrophy, and melancholia, all of which were related to being female and to having "female organs." Others noted that the self-starvation was often accompanied by melancholia, or sadness, as we sometimes see today alongside anorexia. Therefore, they theorized that the self-starvation may have been part of a suicidal intention. Another popular explanation during the time was that anorexia was due to "chlorosis," a name given to patients who had a greenish tinge to their skin, along with other symptoms such as lack of appetite, decreased energy, headache, shortness of breath, anemia, and amenorrhea (Bemporad 1996). In 1840, Thomas Laycock, a physician from York, commented on the relationship between anorexia and hysteria:

> *In no chronic disease is this symptom so constant and so strongly marked as in hysteria . . . Nothing is more true than that a hysterical girl will live and look fat on an incredibly small quantity of food, and that exclusively vegetable* (Laycock 1840).

THE FOREFATHERS OF A NEW DISEASE: ANOREXIA NERVOSA

As with any great discovery, there are many people who do the research and find clues leading up to the discovery but don't make that final leap. Such is the case with anorexia nervosa. Although Sir William Gull and Dr. Charles Laségue are credited with being the first to describe anorexia nervosa as a unique illness, many other well-known physicians, including William Stout Chipley (in 1859), Pierre Briquet (in 1859), and Louis-Victor Marcé (in 1860) did the background work. They were among the first to note that self-starvation was a symptom of a disease, although they did not take that final step, describing self-starvation as a disease of its own. Without their work, Gull and Laségue may not have been able to make their discovery.

William Stout Chipley

William Stout Chipley (1810–1880) was the chief medical officer at the Eastern Lunatic Asylum of Kentucky. He was the first American physician who, in 1859, published in *The American Journal of Insanity* descriptions of self-starvation in American insane asylums. He referred to their fasting as "sitophobia" and thought it was one symptom of several different types of insanity. He said that sitophobia in the insane was caused either by organic or by moral causes. While the organic cause was usually a digestive problem, moral causes included those who feared the food was poisoned and those who would not eat for a supernatural or divine reason (van Deth and Vandereycken 2000).

Chipley then discussed another group of patients who refused food and tended toward hysteria. Typically, they were adolescent girls who had been brought to the asylum by their parents because they refused to eat. Usually their family physician recommended it after unsuccessfully trying to prevent weight loss and its accompanying medical complications. This group arrived at the asylum in a state of emaciation and physical deterioration. Chipley thought these girls differed from previous sitophobes because, although they admitted that eating distressed them, they denied that it was due to any special powers or divine inspiration. Chipley recognized that this group of girls felt that refraining from eating was an accomplishment that made them special and unique and, furthermore, that it was a way to attract attention, sympathy, and power from family and friends. He also observed that these girls came from educated, rational middle-class families. Chipley viewed these girls as manipulative with a "vicious habit" of not eating, and he thought that they indeed needed to enter the asylum for forced feeding and moral treatment which, hopefully, could save their lives (Silverman 1983).

Pierre Briquet

Pierre Briquet (1796–1881) was an internist who was the head of a ward in a Parisian hospital. While performing research on another disease, he observed that there were several hysterical patients who had symptoms which were similar to one another but different from the "typical hysteric." Although Briquet thought that all types of hysteria came from the "affective" part of the brain, he called this second type of hysteria "hyperaesthesia of digestion" or "gastralgia," because one of the symptoms they had in common was stomach pains. Other symptoms he observed in this group, which mainly consisted of adolescent females (he noted that males can also have hysteria in the ratio of 1:20), included irregular menstruation, chlorosis—a green hue to the skin due to iron deficiency anemia, and a gradual decrease in appetite. They also developed an aversion toward ordinary food, sometimes having an attack of hysteria if they ate a particular food, and acquired a strange appetite. Briquet observed that, no matter what type of food aversion they had, it always appeared to be influenced by unpleasant experiences and emotions. He recommended pleasant experiences to decrease or resolve this type of hysteria. Along with several of his assistants, Briquet gathered data on 430 hysterical patients over a 10-year period. He published his observations in 1859 in his book, *Traité Clinique et Thérapeutique de l'Hystérie*, although it didn't receive much attention until many years later (Vandereycken and van Deth 1994). Some of the observations he noted are still relevant today in those who have anorexia nervosa.

Louis-Victor Marcé

Louis-Victor Marcé (1828–1864) was a French physician who directed a large asylum in Paris. Some say he was the first to actually publish a modern medical account of anorexia nervosa. In 1859 he delivered a speech to the medical society of Paris, where he discussed a group of young girls who, around the time of puberty, "arrive at a delirious conviction that they cannot or ought not to eat" and who were oppositional and obsessive about food—characteristics seen in modern-day anorexics. He disagreed with the common idea of his era that these symptoms were due to a disturbance of the stomach. Instead, he surmised that a nervous disturbance around the time of menarche may have led to a "partial insanity" (Silverman 1987b).

During his speech, Marcé discussed some difficult cases and warned other physicians that relapses were common among these girls, and that some could actually die from malnutrition. Marcé noted physiologic changes that accompanied the self-starvation, including constipation, loss of monthly menstruation, and sleeplessness. His treatment recommendations, like Chipley's, were to remove the girls from their families and force feed them. He suggested gradually increasing the amount of food given each day and, if the patient refused, he encouraged methods such as intimidation or force feeding through an esophageal probe (Bemporad 1996). Even if they appear to have recovered, he emphasized the need to follow them for a long period of time because of their risk of relapsing.

Marcé gave two interesting case reports, including that of Mademoiselle X, who developed a dislike for food soon after she had reached menarche. She decreased her food intake until she was only taking a few spoonfuls of soup a day, although reluctantly. Otherwise, she was healthy and appeared content with her small daily intake. With time she became emaciated, could barely stand, and always felt cold. Although she was aware of how sick she had become, she could not force herself to eat, especially when she was with her family. Marcé removed her from her home and put her in someone else's care.

Over the next two months she increased her food intake and had basically recovered, so she returned home. However, because she continued to have some strange eating patterns and behaviors, Marcé was not confident that she was totally cured and was concerned that she might relapse. Her final outcome is not known (Bell 1985).

Sir William Gull

Sir William Gull (1816–1890) was a well-educated and renowned London physician and consultant who became the physician for Queen Victoria and her family. His accomplishments are remarkable. He was a fellow and member of the elite Royal College of Physicians and Surgeons, and held jobs in both private practice and at teaching hospitals, where he was exposed to many different types of patients. Although he has been touted by many as the person who first recognized anorexia nervosa as its own disease, separate from other types of wasting diseases, there is ongoing debate as to whether Charles Laségue, a French physician who will be discussed later, was actually the one who should be credited with, or at least share the credit for this discovery (Brumberg 2000).

Gull was very devoted to his patients. Like many other physicians of his era, he wanted to know the facts behind the causes and treatments of illnesses rather than to depend on irrelevant, irrational and outdated hypotheses. In 1868, he was asked to deliver the opening address at the annual meeting of the British Medical Association, where he was to talk about clinical medicine. During the speech, while discussing how he made a diagnosis based on the clinical exam of a patient, he made an indirect reference to emaciated women without mentioning them again during his speech.

> At present our diagnosis is mostly one of inference, from our knowledge of the several organs to particular lesions, thus we avoid the error of supposing the presence of mesenteric disease in young women emaciated to the last degree through hysteric apepsia, by our knowledge of the latter affection, and by the absence of tubercular disease elsewhere (Pearce 2006).

Essentially, Gull was saying that physicians could assume, based on what they already knew about the body, its organs, and other diseases, that some women with emaciation did not have other illnesses commonly diagnosed during that time period, such as hysteric apepsia, tuberculosis, or inherent difficulties as a result of being female.

His address was published in the *Lancet* but he did not discuss self-starvation with regard to women again professionally until 1873, many months after his colleague, Charles Laségue, published a paper, "On Hysterical Anorexia." Soon after Laségue's publication, Gull presented a lecture to the Clinical Society of London on "anorexia hysterica," in which he reminded others that he discussed women with anorexia nervosa during his address to the British Medical Association in 1863 and that the latter paper, published by Laségue, provides further support for his notion that anorexia nervosa is a separate condition. In his lecture, which was later published, Gull makes the following remarks:

> In ... 1868, I referred to a peculiar form of disease occurring mostly in young women, and characterized by extreme emaciation ... At present our diagnosis of this affection is negative, so far as determining any positive cause from which it springs ... The subjects ... are ... chiefly between the ages of sixteen and twenty-three ... The want of appetite is, I believe, due to a morbid mental state ... We might call the state hysterical (Pearce 2006).

In his speech and subsequent paper, Gull differentiated girls between 16 and 23 years of age who simply refused to eat from those who were medically ill or those who had sitophobia. He said that these girls were not thin because they had religious aspirations or were psychotic, but because they were neurotic. He discussed how the term *anorexia nervosa* was better for these girls than the term used previously, *anorexia hysterica*. Gull decided not to use the term *apepsia* because it indicated that the food they ate wasn't well digested, but it was. He preferred the term *anorexia* because it means lack of appetite, and *nervosa* because it indicated the central nervous system was involved, rather than the uterus, which others had thought was directly involved in the development of anorexia. Additionally, by removing the uterus as a prime cause of anorexia nervosa, men could now be included in the diagnosis. Although Gull did acknowledge that Laségue also used the term *anorexia*, he insisted that he thought of it independently of his colleague.

Gull emphasized that anorexia nervosa was different than other illnesses which involved anorexia, or the "lack of an appetite." He observed that clinical symptoms of anorexia nervosa included emaciation, decreases in heart rate and breathing, restlessness despite being weak, and the lack of periods. He also noted that individuals with anorexia nervosa did not complain of feeling sick. Additionally, as a group, they were rather stubborn. Gull did not recommend medications or tonics to treat anorexia nervosa because they didn't work. Instead, he encouraged the family to remove the girl from her home environment and place her elsewhere. In terms of feeds, he suggested a diet of milk, cream, soup, eggs, fish and chicken, to be given every two hours by a trained nurse. He also emphasized warm bed rest, with heat on the spine to aid in the digestion of food. If necessary, he thought that force feeding, possibly through an esophageal tube, was warranted to save the patient (Brumberg 2000).

Charles Laségue

While Gull concentrated on the medical aspects of patients with anorexia nervosa, Charles Laségue emphasized the psychological aspects. Charles Laségue (1816–1883) was a distinguished French psychiatrist who was well-published on a variety of medical topics. He was also chairman of clinical medicine at La Pitié Hospital and co-editor of a leading French journal. He and several colleagues attempted to differentiate groups of patients that were bunched together under the diagnosis of "hysteria." In his articles, Laségue described one type of hysteria that he saw in Victorian middle-class families, which was often related to struggles over eating. He made a connection between emotional struggle or conflicts within these families and the girls' refusal to eat. Laségue developed his theories after observing eight patients, ages 18 to 32 years, and their families. All of these girls were so similar to one another that it was easy to make a diagnosis. Like Gull, Laségue also called these girls "l'anorexie" (anorexic), which means "lack of appetite." And, like Gull, he did not think that digestive issues or matters of the "womb" were responsible for the poor food intake. Yet, unlike Gull, he chose to keep the name "hysterica" rather than "nervosa" because he thought this self-imposed anorexia was due to a problem within the nervous system and with "nervous emotions," referred to as hysteria (Malson 1998).

Laségue defined three stages of "l'anorexie." In the first stage there is an uneasiness, fullness, or suffering after eating. The feeling is sudden, unrelated to what is eaten, and not associated with any medical problems, such as vomiting. The amount of food eaten is gradually decreased, and a variety of reasons are given, such as a fear that the pain will return. At first specific food groups or particular foods are forbidden, but eventually entire meals are skipped. According to Laségue, when the amount of food consumed is miniscule, the disease is established. At first the patient feels fine. The family becomes worried and tries to convince her to begin eating again, either by making her favorite foods or by punishing her for not eating enough. They may try to get her to eat out of feelings of guilt. They tell her that if she loved them she would eat again. Laségue states that when none of this works, the "mental perversion" is in place. In the second stage, the anorexic becomes obsessed with food and with not eating, and she can't think of or talk about anything else. In fact, food or the lack of it becomes the main topic within the entire family.

The girl has become used to the feeling of hunger and is now content with her state of starvation. Her periods become irregular and eventually stop completely, and she may develop constipation that is resistant to medications. In the third stage, emaciation becomes severe and the family becomes very anxious. Other symptoms which may appear if they haven't already are anemia, chronic thirst, dry and pale skin, dizziness, fainting, weakness, and the inability to exercise. Although Laségue wrote that one could die from anorexia, he never personally had a patient who succumbed to the illness. He thought that once the anorexics saw the intense fear of their families, they would gradually begin to eat again (Brumberg 2000).

Although self-starvation has existed for centuries, the reasons for fasting have changed. They have varied from religious devotion to asceticism to possession by the devil. By the nineteenth century, physicians began to recognize and describe groups of patients, mostly women, who refused to eat but otherwise appeared healthy. Since this time period, the number of people with similar symptoms has increased dramatically, particularly for middle-class women in the United States and other Westernized societies.

2

From Sarah Jacobs to Twiggy: Sociocultural and Economic Changes Over the Past Century

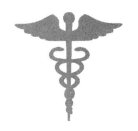

"I won't look at magazines anymore because all I see is tiny, unreasonable people. I feel like I was impressionable before I had anorexia. I followed all the articles in the magazines so I could look just like the models."

—Ari

Western society has changed enormously over the past 150 years—economically, politically, culturally, and socially. Overall, these changes have been of greater magnitude for women than for men, although they have also occurred in males. American culture has transformed from one which placed great importance on people's inner values to a culture which values superficial beauty and thinness, particularly in women. Some of these changes have occurred because of the influence of the media and entertainment industries. They have increasingly focused on superficial beauty and have presented female role models whose appearance is almost, if not entirely impossible to emulate. In addition, other factors, such as more relaxed attitudes toward sex and sexuality, have also contributed to the middle-class transformation from a focus on inner, moral values to more superficial ones.

FROM HOMEMAKER TO TEACHER: POLITICAL AND EDUCATIONAL CHANGES FOR WOMEN

Many of the major changes that we see today began in the latter half of the 1800s. During this period, a typical middle-class wife was the care-taker of her family and home, often with the help of one or more serv-ants. Due to their new roles within society, these women had more free time, so they were able to explore the culture and arts. In addition, such families had more disposable income than previously, which they were more likely to spend on vacation, sports, and music (MacKenzie 2001). Like men, many European and American women were developing grand ideas. These women wanted improved education, employment, and political equality. While some men thought women didn't need an education to be successful in their role as homemaker, others believed that women should be given the same opportunities that men had. Eventually, higher educa-tion was offered to women. Secondary schools and colleges were opened specifically for females, such as Mount Holyoke College in Massachusetts, which began offering a four-year curriculum in 1862. In 1876, the London School of Medicine allowed women to register as doctors. The number of American women attending college increased from 21% in 1870 to 40% in 1910 (Solomon 1985). By the twentieth century, the number of women graduates, and the percentage of those holding nontraditional jobs changes considerably. In the 1920s the number of girls graduating high school exploded. By the mid-1980s, the percentage of females graduating from college climbed to 49%. Although about 70% of women who graduated from a woman's college in 1915 worked, most of the jobs were traditional, such as secretaries and teachers. By the mid-1980s, however, women had earned 49% of all master's degrees and 33% of all doctoral degrees (Chafe 1992).

Along with educational equality, some women also demanded political equality. They wanted the right to vote. In the 1860s, many women's rights organizations were formed to fight for this cause (Chafe 1992). Some women used extreme tactics to publicize their position on these issues, such as set-ting fire to mailboxes, chaining themselves to railings, setting off bombs, and even participating in hunger strikes. Women who starved themselves were often jailed and force fed. As a result of their activism, women finally won the right to vote in 1920. By the early twentieth century, females also began to demand equal pay for performing the same jobs as men. It was not until 1963 that the Equal Pay Act was passed in Congress (Farah and Karls 2001).

THE TRANSFORMATION FROM INNER TO OUTER BEAUTY

The social and cultural changes which have occurred over the past century have been vast. During the Victorian Era, many women were concerned about their inner beauty or their moral character. Historian Joan Jacobs Brumberg, who analyzed diaries of adolescent girls during the nineteenth and twentieth centuries, found that teens in the 1800s rarely mentioned their physical characteristics, but instead focused on improving their values and manners. Organizations and clubs, such as the Girl Scouts, were set up to focus on spiritual and moral aspirations and to teach good values. However, these values began to change during the early twentieth century. As the middle class continued to grow and more families were able to afford nonessentials, such as fancy clothes and jewelry, they started to notice the way they and others looked and dressed. Their appearance took on greater significance. In addition, with the financial ability to purchase items such as mirrors and scales, there were more ways to evaluate their own looks. Whereas previously women only weighed themselves at county fairs and doctors' offices, they could now do it as often as they wanted in the privacy of their own homes. Awareness of their own bodies and that of others increased further when, in the early 1900s, the first set of healthy weights, based on height and sex, were published. People now had a means by which to compare themselves to others with similar body types (Brumberg 1997).

PETTICOATS TO FLAPPERS: CHANGES IN WOMEN'S CLOTHING

Women's fashions went through a dramatic transition during the beginning of the twentieth century, from clothes which covered practically every part of their body to clothes which were more form fitting and exposed a fair amount of skin. During the Victorian Era, women wore a corset to attain an hourglass figure. Their outer dress consisted of multiple layers of petticoats, long skirts, frills, and lace. They also often wore a rigid hoop skirt to hold their multiple layers. Neither their legs nor their ankles were ever exposed, even in the middle of the summer. Even the Gibson Girls, the name given to the glamorous women illustrated by Charles Dana Gibson in magazines in the late 1800s, wore clothing which covered almost their entire bodies (Figure 2.1). They had long hair, pulled up high in the back and covered by a large, wide-brimmed hat; a tight collar with large, full sleeves; a small waist with a boned, laced corset; many petticoats; bloomers; and stockings (Rollin 1999).

By the beginning of the twentieth century, two important changes took place with regard to clothing styles. The first is attributed to Paul Poiret

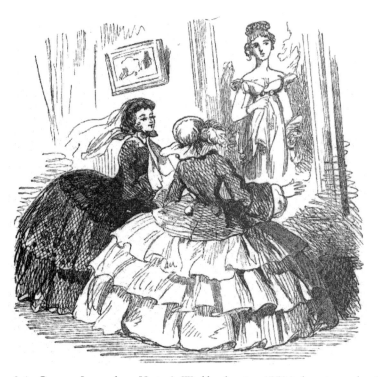

Figure 2.1. Cartoon Image from *Harper's Weekly*, showing 1850s' changing styles. This cartoon, from the July 11, 1857 issue of *Harper's Weekly*, shows how women's fashions changed during the Victorian Era from those of previous time periods. The Victorian style included multiple layers of clothing from head to toe, where very little skin was exposed. [Photo Courtesy of National Library of Congress]

(1879–1944), a well-known Parisian fashion designer, who revolutionized clothing fashions in Europe and the United States by designing a slim, straight-style dress. Unlike previous styles, this one looked best on small-breasted, thin women who had long narrow hips. To ensure that it fit right, however, a woman had to forego her corset for a girdle. Clothing styles which emerged after this prototypical dress continued to have the French influence, with increased emphasis on the slim, small-busted, and narrow-waisted woman (Cunningham 2003). This is evident in "the flapper style" dress, which was introduced in the 1920s. For this dress to fit right, a woman not only had to be thin, but she also had to use a flattening brassiere rather than one that lifted up and accentuated her breasts (Figure 2.2). Additionally, the hemline ended just below the knee, so more leg was exposed than ever before (Brumberg 2000).

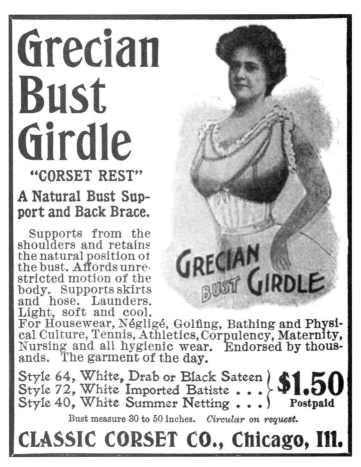

Figure 2.2. Advertisement for a "Bust Girdle" in 1901. This advertisement illustrates the beginning of a new era, where undergarments are produced in factories rather than at home and where women have to fit into specific sizes rather than have garments made to fit their shapes. The girdle advertised above, while still covering a large part of the torso, is less cumbersome than undergarments worn during the Victorian Era. [Photo courtesy of Wikimedia]

The second significant change that took place around the turn of the century was that, for the first time, a woman's body had to fit into her dress rather than the other way around. Previously, women usually made their own dresses, and each was measured and made to fit the individual body measurements of that particular woman. In the early 1900s, however, dresses began to be mass-produced, and by the 1920s, standard sizes were introduced. Not only did a woman's body have to fit into the outfit, but she had a number with

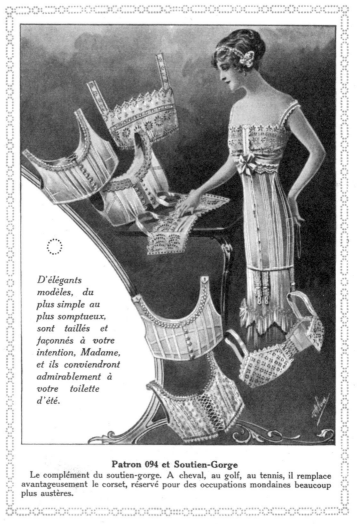

D'élégants
modèles, du
plus simple au
plus somptueux,
sont taillés et
façonnés à votre
intention, Madame,
et ils conviendront
admirablement à
votre toilette
d'été.

Patron 094 et Soutien-Gorge
Le complément du soutien-gorge. A cheval, au golf, au tennis, il remplace
avantageusement le corset, réservé pour des occupations mondaines beaucoup
plus austères.

Figure 2.3. Advertisement for Brassieres and Slips in a French Publication. The woman in this illustration, most likely from the 1920s, is much slimmer and flat-chested than those seen in advertisements from previous years. The brassieres she is advertising are sexier, expose more body, and are made for thinner, flat-chested women. [Photo courtesy of Wikimedia]

which to compare her body size to that of others. Women who were very over-weight may not have been able to find a dress that fit them. The same occurred with brassieres, which were rapidly replacing corsets (Figure 2.3). Instead of being made at home, they also were being mass-produced with standard sizing. Again, women were given a number by which to compare themselves to others.

This process was understandably difficult for conservative, private females who had to go to a store, have measurements taken by an unknown person, try to fit into a premade shape and size, and then buy the brassiere. Seemingly benign cultural changes such as these have contributed over time to making our society more conscious and aware of our body size and shape. They have also made it easier to compare our bodies to those of others and perhaps more likely to compete for a "better" body size.

FROM DRESS SIZING TO DIETING

Standard dress sizes, along with the discovery of the food calorie and nutritional value of foods at the end of the nineteenth century, are some of the factors which led to increased dieting among middle-class Americans (Hargrove 2006). Issues surrounding food were already an integral part of society for eighteenth century middle- and upper-class women. They refrained from eating too much and avoided certain foods for fear that they would look bad in front of others or would appear to have a sexual appetite. Even some teens were beginning to think that they needed to control their weight. In the late 1880s, a group of French schoolgirls competitively dieted with each other, many by drinking vinegar and trying to take in the fewest calories (Habermas 2005).

People learned that certain foods were healthful while others weren't, that all food had calories, and that they should only consume a certain number of calories each day to maintain a healthy weight. Although the overall concern in the early 1900s was that of underweight children, some middle-class women began to worry that they weighed too much and needed to control their food intake. By the early 1920s, doctors agreed that women needed to control their weight, and they began to discuss the medical problems associated with being overweight. During the same period, standard tables of "average" weights were replaced by "desirable" weights.

Although there are accounts of people dieting before the twentieth century, it wasn't common until the 1920s, when weight, particularly "overweight," made its way into the public eye. Lulu Hunt Peters, a physician from California, was partially responsible for the increased awareness about dieting. In 1918, she published the first best-selling diet book about weight control, calories, and weight loss. In her book, Peters gave advice about dieting and taught people about sources of calories and daily caloric requirements. She urged others to think about every piece of food as a specific number of calories and encouraged them to think about whether they really needed those extra calories. Dr. Peters also wrote about how she had been obese but lost a significant amount of weight, and she described how she did it. As can be seen in the excerpt from her book, her eating habits were not entirely healthful. She discussed periods of partial fasting, relying on coffee to make her feel full. She also paid no attention to nutritional content.

> I stopped going to the breakfast table. I kept some canned milk and coffee in my room, and made me two cups of coffee. For lunch I ate practically what I wanted, limiting myself to one slice of bread or one potato (we had no butter), with fruit for dessert. For dinner I came down only when the dessert was being served, and had a share of that with some coffee (Peters 1918).

THE SKIN AS A SYMBOL OF SUPERFICIAL BEAUTY

Along with the other transformations from inner to outer beauty came the advent of skin care. In the Victorian Era, acne was thought to be an outward sign of sexual promiscuity. This was very stressful for a teenager who had a lot of pimples, and embarrassing for her family because sex and sexuality were not admirable qualities in women. Teens often used many different types of astringents and chemicals in attempts to get rid of their pimples, although they didn't always work. With the arrival of mirrors in homes, teens were frequently reminded about their facial imperfections. Additional reminders came from mothers, who wanted to help their daughters become acne-free. If home remedies didn't help, mothers brought them to doctors. Unfortunately, these visits had a negative effect on teens because it made them think that their pimples really were a problem. Rather than reassure families, physicians sometimes made matters worse. By the mid-1900s physicians were recommending that teens make appointments as soon as they saw even a small pimple forming. Physicians were concerned that pimples could cause unsightliness, in addition to poor self-esteem. Since middle-class women did not want to be responsible for their children's lack of self-esteem, they followed the doctors' advice. Pimples, or the lack of them, became so important that, according to Brumberg in her book, *The Body Project*, at least one family decided to pay for acne treatment in lieu of sending a daughter to college. Her family was willing to forego an entire education to improve their daughter's looks, another sign that appearance was becoming of paramount importance to Americans.

Middle-class society also found other ways to demonstrate their new fascination with appearance when many women began to use facial makeup. By the 1920s, women were using multiple products, including powders, rouge, lipstick, and eyelash curlers. They preferred bright colors, including deep red for the lips and turquoise on the eyelids; and their eyes were heavily outlined. One of the first beauty companies to market makeup for the average female was already promoting an unrealistic idea of how all American women should look when they came up with the public relations slogan, "Every girl could look like a movie star by using Max Factor® make-up." Max Factor® was already setting up women to fail. In addition to makeup, women also tried to improve their appearance through changes in their hairstyles. Between 1922 and 1927, the number of hair salons in New York City grew from 750 to 3,500 (Rollin 1999).

SEXUALITY TRANSFORMS FROM PERSONAL TO IMPERSONAL

American society was also transforming from one that rarely discussed personal issues to one that not only discussed them, but also became increasingly comfortable with them. For example, since the beginning of the twentieth century, teens have become much more at ease and are more willing to discuss sexuality and sexual behaviors. In addition, sexual behaviors are also more acceptable today than they were at the turn of the century. Their acceptance, however, has led to increased pressure to look "sexy," placing the emphasis once again on the teen's outer appearance. These new attitudes did not occur overnight, but changed gradually. The transformation began around the 1920s, when some mothers started to discuss previously taboo subjects, such as puberty and menarche. Physicians also began to discuss personal topics which were related to a teenager's health. In addition, doctors started to ask gender-specific questions and perform full examinations. During the same time period, teens were becoming more sexually promiscuous. They wanted to distinguish themselves from people of the previous generation, and increased sexuality was one way to do it. Women began to flaunt themselves and engage in behaviors they never would have considered 30 years earlier. This is one reason sexual experimentation increased in the 1920s. It was not uncommon for teens and young adults to kiss and "pet" in the back of an automobile (Rollin 1999). Finally, companies contributed to the increased comfort level regarding personal issues by producing and advertising products which had previously been made in the privacy of one's home. This included sanitary napkins in the 1920s and tampons in the 1930s.

Experimentation and approval of sexual behaviors increased further in the second half of the century. According to Brumberg, the diaries of teen girls over the past few decades have become much more explicit and detail-oriented in terms of sexual behaviors, and less romantic than the diaries of the earlier 1900s. The increased comfort with and acceptance of sexuality is evident in the doctor's office where, since the 1960s, doctors have been prescribing oral contraceptives as a form of birth control to unwed teens. In American society, any form of birth control can be given to a teen without a parent's knowledge or consent. Because of all these changes, teens are forced to behave like adults and deal with mature topics at ages far younger than previously, and at earlier ages than what is reasonable. The fact that girls are reaching menarche younger than ever before, less than age $12^1/_2$ years, has led to a further decrease in the age at which girls must deal with such topics.

Not only are teens supposed to think like adults, but many expect them to look and act like adults. Nowadays, it is common to see ten- and eleven-year-old girls wearing makeup, dangling earrings, high-heeled shoes, shirts with bras and stomachs that are exposed, and shorts that barely cover their upper thighs. They have spent a lot of time and money to look good, so any imperfection can be a major disaster (YWCA n.d.). Many are quick to make an appointment with a dermatologist if they see the slightest eruption on their face. If their friends are thinner than they are, they feel fat.

Sometimes, parents accentuate the problem. For instance, they may want their children to look perfect. If they see their child with a pimple, they may recommend a face cream or make an appointment with a dermatologist. They worry that imperfect skin will have an effect on their child's self-esteem. If their child's teeth aren't perfectly aligned, they whisk them off to the orthodontist for braces. Once their child is old enough, often by age 9 or 10, they may begin the search for designer clothes. Also, parents may role model this unrealistic, intense desire for superficial perfection. Parents, mostly moms, often complain about their own bodily imperfections, whether it is their weight, wrinkles, cellulite, hair, or some other superficial flaw. Instead of quietly accepting natural changes that come with age, adult women undergo surgical procedures in hopes of improving their looks or reclaiming their younger years. This might include a tummy tuck, plastic surgery, liposuction, or botox injections. Or it might be in the form of gastric bypass surgery or breast augmentation. The list is endless. And their children are watching. They are seeing that thin, beautiful, and sexy is the goal for which they must aim. A recent study, "Beauty at Any Cost," documented that 7 billion dollars a year is spent on cosmetics alone. In 2007, 11.7 million cosmetic surgical and nonsurgical procedures were completed, an almost 500% increase from 10 years earlier. In 2008, females ages 18 to 24 years approved more of cosmetic surgical procedures than any other age group, with 69% thinking it was a good idea (YWCA n.d.)

All of these changes are taking a toll on teens. They are receiving the message that sex and sexuality are no big deal. These days, puberty, menarche, and periods are seen as major steps toward independence and another step away from the core family. Young teens are relying on friends instead of parents to help them deal with personal problems, especially when it pertains to sex and sexual behavior. Yet neither they nor their peers are emotionally or cognitively mature enough to handle some of the issues with which they must deal. Some experts believe that sexuality is intricately tied into anorexia nervosa. Anorexia often begins around puberty, when teens are forced to think of themselves as adults with adult sexual characteristics and increased body fat; and when individuals must learn to deal with complicated "adult" issues. Those who develop anorexia may be trying to avoid all of these issues for a variety of reasons, including sexual repression and increased control over their lives (Gordon 2000).

EFFECT OF EARLY MASS MEDIA ON WOMEN

Over the past 150 years, both mass media and the entertainment industry have had a significant effect on society's obsession with superficial beauty and the desire to be thin. The transformation began in the late 1800s and early 1900s, when many middle-class women had more leisure time and were able to afford a daily newspaper. During this time period, the circulation of both newspapers and magazines increased significantly during the end of the nineteenth century. In 1873, New York began to publish a daily paper with illustrations, and by 1878 they had the first full-page newspaper advertisements. Unlike earlier magazines, which were read mainly by the upper class, women's magazines which started publication around the turn of the century catered to the needs and desires of middle-class women. The six largest magazines for women, *Delineator, McCall's, Ladies' Home Journal, Woman's Home Companion, Good Housekeeping,* and *Pictorial Review,* focused on topics which could help middle-class women with their homemaking abilities. They published articles which gave advice and guidance about beauty, etiquette, and fashion, sometimes providing a variety of views on a particular topic. Advertising became more important and companies targeted their products toward women because they were the ones who purchased them. This included not only items for the home, but also skin care products and makeup. During the early twentieth century, additional products were purchased after physicians began to urge women to improve their outer appearance by dieting, exercising, and using good hygiene (Zuckerman 1998).

As American women became more concerned with their appearance in the early 1900s, so did society as a whole. Through the entertainment industry, Americans were exposed much more often to beautiful women whose looks were difficult for most girls and women to attain. Beauty pageants, which became very popular, focused mainly on outer appearance and included a bathing suit competition. Models were used for newspapers and magazines. Furthermore, the image and appearance of silent screen stars changed. They became thinner, wore a lot of makeup, and began to expose more of their arms and legs than previously. Well-known stars, such as Clara Bow and Joan Crawford, were viewed as sex symbols. These stars, along with others, such as Annette Kellerman, who had also been a professional swimmer, became role

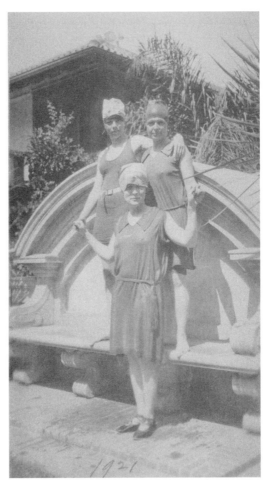

Figure 2.4. Three Women in Bathing Suits in 1921. By the 1920s, women were showing much more skin in public than even 20 years earlier. In this photo, women wore bathing suits which went down to the knee but exposed the entire lower leg and upper arms. [Photo courtesy of The Bancroft Library, University of California, Berkeley]

models for the new, modern woman. Kellerman brought the first above-the-knee bathing suits to the United States (Figure 2.4).

Women compared almost every part of their body to those of others who were wearing the same type of modern suit. Kellerman strongly encouraged women to exercise and eat well so they could maintain a fit figure. The reason, she said, was because a poor figure might lead to the inability to find or keep a good husband. Women bought into these new ways of living. They wanted to separate themselves from the ultra-conservatives of the Victorian Era.

MASS MEDIA AND THE TRANSFORMATION
OF THE IDEAL WOMAN

A large part of what we perceive to be the ideal woman today comes from what we see and read in the mass media and entertainment industry. The media has been responsible for advertising and promoting an unrealistic picture of the perfect woman. Barbie is a prime example of how ridiculously women are portrayed. She is the stereotypical blonde-haired, blue-eyed beauty with the perfect body who, if she were made into a life-sized woman, would be 5 feet 6 inches tall, 110 pounds, with a 39-inch bust, an 18-inch waist and 33-inch hips—which is impossible. She would actually have to crawl on her hands and knees because she would fall over if she tried to stand up. She would certainly meet the weight criterion for anorexia nervosa. Real-life beauties, such as models, *Playboy* centerfolds, and Miss America pageant contestants are also becoming thinner and are setting a standard that is difficult to emulate, in addition to the fact that it is incredibly unhealthy (Brumberg 2000). The average runway model is 5'9" and 110 pounds, which is even worse than Barbie in terms of how much one weighs for their particular height. Twenty years ago a runway model's average weight was 8% lower than expected for their height; today it is more than 20% lower than what is optimal for their height. In 1960, the average weight of *Playboy* models was 9% below average; by 1978 it was 16% below. Miss America contestants weighed 12% less than the national average before 1970 and 15% below average after 1970, again meeting the weight criterion for anorexia nervosa. Yet when surveyed, many of these women said that they were still not at their desirable weight. In addition to the decrease in their weight, these women have also become less curvaceous. Since the 1960s, the average bust and hip sizes in *Playboy* models, runway models, actresses, and Miss America pageant contestants have all decreased (Turner et al. 1997).

By choosing the specific types of articles and advertisements they publish, magazines, in particular, have helped create and perpetuate the stereotypical

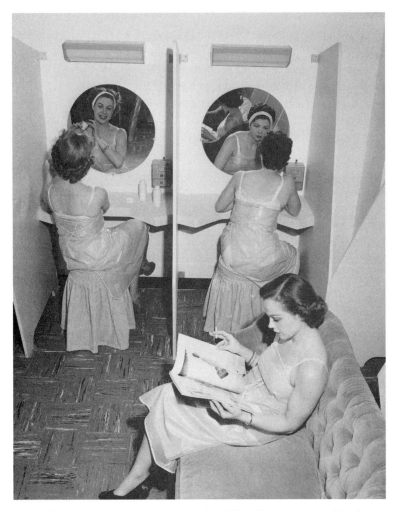

Figure 2.5. Women Putting on Makeup in the 1950s. The women in this photograph, taken in 1952, are reapplying their makeup and freshening up at the "Pamper House" in New York. [Photo courtesy of AP images, Ed Ford]

ideal woman and an environment where looks are much more important than other attributes, such as intellectual abilities. The popularity of magazines, books, and newspapers increased in the early 1900s when women's education and literacy rates increased. In the 1940s, when dieting and weight control became very popular, women's magazines ran articles on this topic not only for adults but also for teens. The *Ladies Home Journal* advised teens to become "beauty conscious" at a young age, and teens were told to "resist the three

S's: sundaes, sodas, and second helpings" (Brumberg 2000). According to several studies, the basic content of women's magazines has not changed significantly over the past 30 years. The basic messages are that every normal female will (or should) get married, and that they can increase their chances by being less competent, more passive, thin, and beautiful. Currently, women's magazines have 10.5 times more advertisements and articles concerning weight loss than men's magazines (Media Awareness Network, "Beauty and Body Image in the Media" n.d.). And, over three-quarters of the front covers of women's magazines have at least one message about how to change a woman's appearance, whether it is through diet, exercise, changes in hairstyle, or cosmetic surgery (Zuckerman 1998).

Vogue and *Cosmopolitan*, two popular women's magazines which have been published since the late 1800s, frequently have articles about sex, fashion, and relationships. In the 1950s, they often ran articles on how to actively change one's looks. A 1957 article in *Vogue* is a prototypical commentary of the times. It was titled "How to Look Like a Beauty," and made women feel ugly and as if they actually had to change their looks if they didn't want to be offensive to others. In the article it discussed how some women "hide their good looks behind frowzy hair, fat, badly-chosen spectacles, and dreary clothes." The author continued by commenting that if a woman wanted to look like a beauty she could, even if she didn't have "inherited good looks." The readers were warned that looking good could take much time, effort, and money, and there was a strong suggestion that "if her hair is a natural disaster, she goes to the very best hairdresser and gets the very best advice as well as the very best work that she can." This includes dyeing the hair, getting a permanent, or having hair straightened (Rollin 1999).

The first magazine targeted for teens was *Seventeen*, which began publication in 1944, and was written for girls ages 12 to 24 years. Its focus was fashion, physical beauty, entertainment, and romance. Initially it ran articles about teens' appearances, advertised the latest clothing styles among middle-class girls, and provided advice on topics such as how to be popular and pimple-free. It did and still does have many advertisements targeted to teens which insinuate that, by using a certain product, they will become popular and self-confident. According to Brumberg, in the mid-1940s *Seventeen* ran articles on nutrition, but by the end of the decade the articles were more specifically about controlling weight and refraining from binge eating. By the 1950s, diet foods came onto the scene and they were advertised along with statements such as "Nobody Loves a Fat Girl" (Brumberg 2000). Nowadays, the magazine focuses on such topics, sending a message that teens should be concerned with their physical appearance and with pleasing a male, even if it means neglecting academics; and that beauty and thinness will lead to popularity and male companionship. *Seventeen* also deals with sexual issues, which in earlier publication years meant articles about dating and self-development but now means frank discussions about sexual issues. Additionally, there is a place where teens can get answers to questions they are too embarrassed to talk to their parents about (Schlenker, Caron, and Halteman 1998). In summary, it is likely that a reader of this magazine is receiving the message that she must not only look, but also act like the models featured in the magazine. In addition, she is receiving information and being given opportunities to become more independent and responsible for her own actions before she is emotionally mature enough.

For decades, the media has focused on makeup, clothing, and weight loss through dieting as a way to improve a woman's appearance. More recently, the media has also begun to make recommendations for men. Their focus has been on exercise, body building, and extreme weight control through sports such as wrestling, running, and rowing. This has led to an explosion of health and fitness magazines geared toward men, such as *GQ, Men's Vogue, Men's Fitness, and Men's Health*. The articles and advertisements in these magazines have historically stressed improving muscle and body shape rather than dealing with actual weight in males because this is what our society values in males. Recently, however, there has been an increase in the number of advertisements and articles for men regarding dieting, although the media continues to emphasize body building over calorie restriction for males, while the opposite is true for females (Hill 2004). As with females, males in our society are now spending more time and money on their appearance, and they are willing to go to extreme measures to develop a better outer appearance. There are now pectoral (chest) and calf muscular implants available for men. Males are having plastic surgery, such as face lifts, and botox injections to make themselves look younger (Cohn 2000). Additionally, skin care and cosmetic companies, which previously only marketed to women, are now advertising items specifically for men, and they are getting the message.

TWIGGY COMES INTO THE SPOTLIGHT

Given all the changes that occurred regarding mass media and popular culture, it was only a matter of time before the world's first supermodel came onto the scene. It happened in 1966 with the discovery of "Twiggy," who at 16 years of age and a height of 5'7" weighed a mere 90 pounds and looked more like a young boy than a teen girl (Figure 2.6). Whereas a basal metabolic index (BMI) (a calculation involving height and weight) below 18.5 is considered underweight, hers was 14. She became an idol for millions of teenage girls and

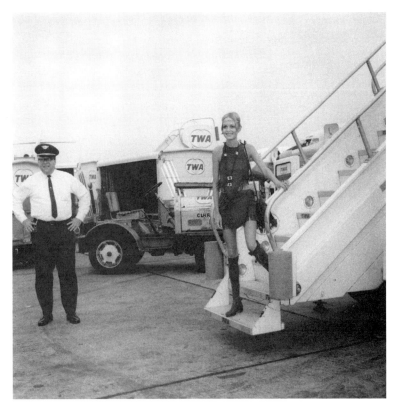

Figure 2.6. The Model, Twiggy. This photo is of the first true supermodel, Twiggy, age 17, as she arrives in New York in August 1967. She was 5'7" and weighed 90 pounds. Many teens wanted to emulate her looks and physique. [Photo courtesy of AP images, TWA]

was on the cover of several magazines, including *Vogue*, *Mod*, and *Mod Teen World*, and was frequently featured in *Elle*. Her popularity and success as a role model significantly influenced the rest of the entertainment industry, which has helped create an unrealistic image of the ideal woman.

THE PUBLIC LEARNS ABOUT ANOREXIA

During the "Twiggy" era, the American public began to learn about anorexia. At first they were misinformed and didn't understand what it truly meant to have anorexia. They couldn't understand how individuals could starve themselves and why they didn't just begin to eat again once they realized they were getting too thin. In the late 1960s and early 1970s, newspapers and magazines

began to publish articles about anorexia nervosa and, at the same time, to educate the public about the illness anorexia nervosa. In 1969, the *Port Arthur
News* ran an article, "Teen Age Danger—Dieting until Death!" In the article,
anorexia nervosa was defined as an "aversion to food caused by psychological
hang-ups so strong even hunger cannot overcome it." The author described an
18-year old who wanted to look like her modeling idol, Twiggy, and ended up
dying as a 45-pound skeleton. In an attempt to educate the public, they noted
that anorexia is far more serious than "high-strung absence of hunger pangs"
("Teen Age Danger"1969). Another article, which ran in *The New York Times*
in 1974, "Children Who Starve Themselves" (Blum 1974), discussed how "anorexics look like gorgeous waifs, but they may be simply trying not to grow up."
The article reassured parents that they could readily recognize anorexia nervosa
in their children because "they take almost no nourishment and the physical
changes are dramatic." But it also states that the disease could end in death.

> No one can prove it—there are no statistics—but the incidence of anorexia
> nervosa, once thought an extraordinarily rare condition, seems to be up. Sim-
> ply described, anorexia nervosa is willful self-starvation, sometimes to the point
> of death (Blum 1974).

The following year, an article called "The Self-Starvers" was published in
Time Magazine.

> At 17, Susan looked alarmingly emaciated, with sunken eyes and fragile,
> sticklike arms and legs. Though she was 5 ft. 5 in. tall, she weighed only
> 70 lbs. and scorned all but the tiniest morsels of food. Amazingly, Susan
> believed herself to be too fat and maintained a frenzied level of physical exercise
> to help keep any weight off her scrawny frame ("The Self-Starvers" 1975).

Anorexia was labeled "the starvation disease," or "the Twiggy Syndrome"
and the author wrote that it is a bizarre emotional disorder that is rare but has
been occurring more frequently in the past few years. The description of a typical person afflicted with anorexia was that she was mostly female (80%) and
in her early teens, intelligent, ambitious, middle or upper class, and a perfectionist eager to please her parents. Furthermore, the article discusses that the
anorexic suddenly starts to diet and then simply stops eating, sometimes losing
about 50 pounds in a few months. It also discusses how researchers agree that
the disease is purely psychological. Some think it is due to fear of sexuality
and that the anorexic tries to keep herself from becoming a woman. Others
think it is an oral rebellion against over controlling and troubled parents.

In addition to newspaper and magazine articles about anorexia, Dr. Hilde Bruch, one of the world's leading experts on anorexia nervosa, published two books based on 40 years of observation and clinical treatment. The first, *Eating Disorders: Obesity, Anorexia Nervosa, and the Person Within*, published in 1973, was written mainly for the physician and scientist, while the second, *The Golden Cage*, published in 1978, was written for the lay public. In her books, she discusses many of her patients and their struggles with anorexia, including how they developed the illness, physical and psychological characteristics, treatment failures and successes, and family involvement. She also discusses her theories about why those with anorexia develop it and how to best help them. These books significantly increased society's awareness of anorexia. The same year that *The Golden Cage* was published, a fictional book made into a TV movie, *The Best Little Girl in the World*, appeared on the bookshelves (Levenkron 1978). It tells the story of a 15-year-old girl, Kessa, who begins to diet and develops anorexia nervosa. The story, based on actual patients, describes the ordeal Kessa and her family go through as she continues to lose weight, becomes obsessed with food, is increasingly self-absorbed, and ends up in the hospital.

As awareness regarding anorexia has increased, so has the desire to be thin. In fact, it has become an integral part of our society. In 1992, *Working Woman* magazine estimated that, at any given time, 65 million Americans were dieting. The number of diet books in circulation since Dr. Peter's best seller in 1918 has exploded. In 2008, there were over 37,000 books about weight loss, dieting, and weight loss programs for sale on one popular online Web site. The recommendations are as varied as the books. Some authors recommend losing weight by using diet aids, such as *Emily's Vinegar Diet Book*. Others recommend cutting out specific food groups, such as carbohydrates, as seen in the *Low-Carb Diet Book* and *The 3-Hour Diet: How Low-Carb Diets Make You Fat and Timing Makes You Thin*. Some authors tout that losing weight is quick and easy, such as in *The Good Mood Diet: Feel Great While You Lose Weight*, *The Inside-Out Diet: 4 Weeks to Natural Weight Loss*, and *Total Body Health, and Radiance*. Weight loss books have also hit the teen market, with titles such as *The 3-Hour Diet for Teens: Lose Weight and Feel Great in Two Weeks!*; *Slim Down, Shape Up Diets for Teens*; and *Lose It for Life for Teens*.

MEDIA PROVIDES UNREALISTIC ROLE MODELS

Every type of media, whether it is newspaper, magazine, radio, or television, targets its audience through advertisements. Today it is common to see an extremely thin model wearing the latest clothing fashions, modeling a particularly sexy brassiere, using a certain deodorant or anti-pimple product, or eating a diet bar. She is usually placed in a setting where she appears popular and self-confident, supposedly because she is using the intended product. Additionally, she comes across as being very happy and successful. These visual images are influencing individuals, particularly teen girls, both in terms of the products being advertised and the surrounding milieu. Many have internalized the thought that thin is good and fat is bad. In one study, six- to nine-year-olds were asked to characterize people of different body shapes and builds. Both sexes preferred the slender, athletic body, which they labeled as being smart and popular; and disliked the chubby, heavy body types (Hesse-Biber 1997). A very important study done in the late 1990s found that the majority of female students questioned, some as young as fifth grade, were unhappy with their body weight and shape. Girls who read more fashion magazines were more likely to have gone on a diet, tried to lose weight, or exercised because of a magazine article and almost half wanted to lose weight because of a picture in the magazine (Field et al. 1999). In 2003, *Teen* magazine reported that 35% of girls ages six to twelve years have dieted at least once and that 50% to 70% of those who were of normal weight thought they were overweight ("Beauty and Body Image in the Media" n.d.). Another survey found that young girls are more afraid of becoming fat than they are of nuclear war, cancer, or losing their parents (Marcus 2000).

MEDIA PLAYS A ROLE IN THE DEVELOPMENT OF ANOREXIA

Not only has the industry pasted images of thin, perfect women everywhere, but it has also associated thinness and beauty with success and popularity. Likewise, it has promoted the image that being unattractive and overweight is associated with failure and loneliness. As of 1999, the average female television character was 5'7" and weighed about 100 pounds, compared to the average American woman, who at the time was 5'4" and weighed 140 pounds (Marcus 2000). Today, over three-quarters of TV actresses in situational comedies are underweight. Thinner women are often made into the more desirable and successful characters, while heavier actresses are given the less desirable, lonely roles. Additionally, overweight women (and often minimally overweight) receive more negative comments on TV about their bodies than thin women, and 80% of their comments are followed by canned audience laughter ("Beauty and Body Image in the Media" n.d.). Today, many actresses, especially those in the constant limelight, are extremely underweight and some, such as Tracey Gold, Sally Fields, Mary Kate Olsen, and Christina Ricci have admitted to having an eating disorder.

Given that the media presents an unrealistic ideal of the perfect woman, a major focus of research has been whether the media plays a role in increasing our society's obsession with superficial beauty and thinness. Numerous studies have been performed to try to answer this question. They have repeatedly shown that mass media transmits unrealistic thin ideals (Vandereycken 2006), and that being exposed to ideal body types in the media negatively influences how a girl feels about her own body. For example, teens who are exposed to beauty commercials place a greater importance on sex appeal and beauty than those who watch neutral ads (Harrison 1997). Another study found that almost 70% of girls who read magazines admitted that the pictures in them influenced their idea of the perfect body shape (Field et al. 1999). Other studies have demonstrated that exposure to images of thin, young, air-brushed female models is linked to depression, low self-esteem, and the development of unhealthy eating habits in women and girls.

A second important focus of research has been in deciding whether an obsession with thinness and the "perfect woman" can lead to the development of disordered eating or even anorexia nervosa. Once again, studies have demonstrated a connection between media exposure to the ideal body type and eating disorders. Teens who developed eating disorders reportedly read more teen magazines and listened to more teen-related radio programs than those who didn't develop eating problems (Martinez-Gonzalez et al. 2003). A study done in the mid-1990s found that female college students who had disordered eating were more likely to have read magazines and watched TV, especially shows which had thin TV actresses (Harrison and Cantor 1997). In addition, researchers documented that people who watch TV at least three nights a week are 50% more likely to feel fat or overweight. Within this group, two-thirds of the females reported dieting as a result of the TV images, and 15% used vomiting as a weight loss technique (Marcus 2000). Recently, researchers have found that adolescents and young adult women who are attracted to thin media personalities, such as models and TV characters, are more likely to have symptoms of disordered eating, an eating disorder, a drive for thinness, body dissatisfaction, and/or a perfectionist personality than those females with less concern about media personalities (Harrison 1997). All of these studies have consistently demonstrated a connection between media exposure and a drive for thinness, yet researchers are still trying to determine whether the drive for thinness or the attraction to thin media personalities came first.

Although the influence of media on the male's perception of themselves has not been nearly as extreme as it has been on women, there is evidence that this has been changing in recent years. Men are becoming more dissatisfied with their weight and body image. In one study, six- to nine-year-olds were asked to characterize people of different body shapes. Boys responded similarly to girls in that they preferred the thinner body types and disliked the larger ones. In addition, results of a statistical analysis demonstrated that between the years 1972 and 1987, the percentage of men who were dissatisfied with their height increased from 13% to 20%; and the percentage who were dissatisfied with their weight increased from 35% to 41%. Men were also more dissatisfied with their facial appearance in 1987 than in 1972, 20% vs. 10%, respectively (Rollin 1999). As body dissatisfaction is increasing in males, so is the incidence of anorexia nervosa. Current research is finding that the incidence of anorexia in men is increasing from 1 out of 10 to 1 out of 6 (Good 2008).

MEDIA PERSONALITIES ARE MORE LIKELY TO DEVELOP ANOREXIA

Not only has exposure to the media been associated with an increased risk of body dissatisfaction and anorexia in both girls and boys, but media personalities are also much more likely to be diagnosed with it, and some have even died from it. The first and most publicized of these personalities was Karen Carpenter. She was a well-known singer who appeared on magazines and TV shows during the 1970s and early 1980s. She had many Gold and Platinum albums, and also won several Grammy awards. Carpenter developed anorexia in 1967, a time when most people had never heard of it. It began when her doctor put her on a water diet because she was an overweight teen. Before the diet, she weighed 140 pounds. After she reached her target weight, she refused to stop dieting. By 1975 she weighed 80 pounds and was abusing medications daily, including dozens of thyroid pills and laxatives, in an attempt to burn off more calories and rid herself of any food or fluids that were left inside her. She became so weak and malnourished that she collapsed during one of her singing performances. After her collapse, she tried to receive help from several doctors and therapists. While it appeared as if she were on the road to recovery, she had continued to secretly consume large doses of laxatives and thyroid hormone. In 1983, she collapsed and died from cardiac arrest secondary to either chemical imbalances from medicine abuse or from the strain on her heart because of her anorexia (Young n.d.).

The combination of Karen Carpenter's death and increased awareness of anorexia nervosa gave other women in the spotlight the courage to admit that they also had anorexia. One of them was Tracey Gold, an actress from the 1980s' TV sitcom, The Growing Pains. Ms. Gold wrote an autobiographical account of her ordeal with anorexia in Room to Grow: An Appetite for Life. She began her struggle with anorexia nervosa around age nine, and was diagnosed at age eleven. After she received counseling, her weight remained relatively stable until she was nineteen, although it was a struggle. At this point she was an actress for a TV sitcom and, during a long break from taping she gained some weight. On returning, she became the recipient of several "fat jokes" which the writers had added to the script. These comments initiated the beginning of a downward spiral. She began a strict diet, consuming only about 500 calories a day instead of the typical 1,800 calories. She also started to make herself vomit, became obsessed with food, and eventually was hospitalized.

While the entertainment and media industries are largely responsible for providing unrealistic and dangerously thin role models for teens in our society, they are also partially responsible for instigating, encouraging, or, at the very least, ignoring disordered eating and anorexia nervosa in those who work for them. Certain groups are known to support thinner participants than others, including gymnasts, ballet dancers, models, actresses, and professional skaters. For example, a well-known gymnast, Cathy Rigby, was the first American woman to win a medal in a world gymnastics competition and, in 1968, became an Olympic team member. She recalls how her coaches told her that she needed to weigh 90 pounds for her competition. To maintain her desired weight, she often ate only once a day. When she went through puberty, she became even stricter. She discusses that this was a common problem among gymnasts, and that she knows others who used laxatives or self-induced vomiting to maintain their necessary weight. Christy Henrich, another world-class gymnast, died from her anorexia. Just as with Rigby, Heinrich was told by a judge that she needed to lose weight to make the 1992 U.S. Olympic team. She lost almost 30% of her body weight and eventually died from multiple organ system failure. The well-known child actress, Mary-Kate Olsen, has also battled anorexia and has required hospitalization. Heidi Guenther, a ballet dancer, died from anorexia at age twenty-two after she was told that 5'5" and 96 pounds was too "chunky." An American model, Carre Otis, talks about how she did everything from dieting and fasting to using drugs, diet pills, and laxatives for almost seventeen years to maintain her ultra-thin weight. Otis is luckier than other models. In a little over a year, beginning in 2006, four fashion models died from complications due to anorexia. The first was Luisel Ramos, a runway model from Uruguay, who died at age twenty due to heart failure secondary to anorexia. She reportedly subsisted on lettuce and diet drinks. Four months later, Ana Carolina Reston, a Brazilian model who reportedly only ate apples and tomatoes, died from complications of anorexia. She weighed 88 pounds. And a mere two months later, Luisal Ramos' sister Eliana, also a model, died from anorexia. Then, in November 2007, an Israeli fashion model, Hila Elmalich, died weighing less than 60 pounds.

The changes that occurred over the past century have been tremendous. One of the major transformations has been a shift from inner beauty to outer beauty, particularly for women. The media, in an effort to appeal to the modern-day female, has created an image of the perfect woman which is unrealistic and, at times, dangerous. In the journey to become that "perfect woman," some teens, and even adults, develop disordered eating that can develop into anorexia nervosa.

3

Defining Anorexia Nervosa and How It Is Diagnosed

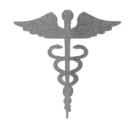

"No matter how thin I was my stomach always bothered me. It was sunken in, yet I always saw it bulging with imaginary fat. All I focused on was diminishing the fat."

—Ari

It has been over a century since anorexia nervosa was first well-described, yet it is still not completely understood how someone develops it or the best way to treat it. In fact, experts do not completely agree on the most accurate way to diagnose this eating disorder and, consequently, its exact definition continues to change. Although there is still much to be discovered, we have already learned a great deal about anorexia, making it easier to identify now than in the past. For instance, it is known that those afflicted with anorexia, mostly females, have a significant weight loss that often goes unnoticed for months or longer by everyone, including family, friends, and physicians. Even the individual who develops it may not realize at first that she is losing so much weight. This illness usually begins as a diet which then takes on a life of its own and leads to a downward spiral, where the initial weight goal has come and gone, and newer, lower target weights are constantly being attained.

CRITERIA USED FOR DIAGNOSING ANOREXIA NERVOSA

Anorexia was described in the 1800s and physicians have been treating it for over a century. Yet, it was not classified as a mental illness until 1980 when the American Psychiatric Association first published the criteria used to diagnose anorexia nervosa in the third edition of its *Diagnostic and Statistical Manual of Mental Disorders* (DSM-III). The DSM is the reference book most commonly used by mental health professionals in the United States and in other parts of the world to classify and diagnose mental and psychiatric conditions. The current manual is the DSM-IV-TR (fourth edition, text revision) (American Psychiatric Association 2000). Another reference book that is used in Europe and other regions to diagnose mental conditions is the *International Statistical Classification of Diseases and Related Health Problems* (ICD-10) (World Health Organization 1992) published by the World Health Organization, an agency of the United Nations that acts as a leading authority on health throughout the world.

According to the DSM-IV-TR, someone who meets all of the following four conditions has anorexia nervosa:

1. A body weight that is consistently 85% or less of what is considered normal for height and age, due to weight loss or lack of weight gain during the adolescent growth spurt
2. An intense fear of gaining weight and becoming fat, despite being underweight
3. Either the denial of or refusal to accept that the low body weight is a problem, excessive influence of body weight and shape on self-worth, and/or a distorted body image perception where they think they are fat even though they are underweight
4. Amenorrhea, or the loss of periods in girls who had begun menstruating, for at least three successive menstrual cycles.

There are two types of anorexia nervosa described in the DSM-IV-TR. The first is the restricting type, where the individual loses weight by severely restricting food intake. Sometimes this is accompanied by abuse of medications. The second is the binge eating/purging type, where someone with the illness will either binge and/or purge during their illness. When someone binges, they eat large quantities of food in a short amount of time. When someone purges, they self-induce vomiting and/or misuse medicines, such as laxatives, diuretics, or enemas, to quickly rid their bodies of food and fluids.

The ICD-10 has its own criteria which it uses to diagnose anorexia nervosa, including all six of the following:

1. Body weight that is consistently 15% or lower than expected for height and age, or a body mass index (BMI, which is a calculation of weight for height) of 17.5 or less; this can be due to weight loss or failure to gain weight during the pubertal growth phase
2. Weight loss that is caused by refusal to eat foods thought to be fattening
3. At least one of the following behaviors is used to lose weight or maintain a low weight: self-induced vomiting, purging, excessive exercise, use of medicines to suppress the appetite or to cause large amounts of fluids to be lost from the body
4. A distorted or unrealistic awareness of one's own body shape and size due to intense and irrational fears of becoming fat, which leads to the desire to stay at a low body weight
5. Evidence of endocrine dysfunction, or abnormal hormone levels which cause amenorrhea in women and impotence or the loss of libido, or sex drive, in males; there may also be changes in hormone levels in either sex, such as growth hormone, cortisol, thyroid hormone, and insulin, which lead to other problems
6. Delay in the onset of puberty in younger females who develop anorexia nervosa.

SIMILARITIES OF THE MAJOR MODELS USED TO DIAGNOSE ANOREXIA

These two classification systems are similar in many ways. Both require a significant amount of weight loss, where the affected individual must weigh 85% or less of what is expected for their specific height and age (ideal body weight or IBW). Often, however, someone with anorexia will only weigh 60% or 70% of their IBW. Both systems also require that the weight loss is due to an extremely restrictive diet due to an intense fear of becoming fat, and not for another unrelated reason. For example, some people don't eat because they are very picky eaters and others don't eat because they have a physical illness that keeps them from feeling hungry. Others who have a mental illness, such as schizophrenia, may have delusional thoughts or hallucinations regarding food and, therefore, are afraid to eat. In all of these situations, however, the person does not limit food intake due to a fear of becoming fat. Therefore, they would not meet all the criteria required to diagnose someone with anorexia.

Individuals with anorexia place extreme limits on the amount and type of food they eat to maximize their weight loss. Most eliminate carbohydrates, such as bread and pasta, and red meat from their diets and concentrate mainly on fruits, vegetables, hot tea, and extremely low fat or nonfat foods. Even then, they limit the intake of these low-calorie items. Their daily caloric intake is far less than the average number needed to maintain one's weight, which is approximately 2,000 calories a day for moderately active older female adolescents and young adults; and around 2,600 calories a day for moderately active older male adolescents and young adults. These values vary with age, height, and activity level. A typical daily diet for an anorexic is often between 500 and 1,000 calories, but can be less. Many examples of daily food logs and caloric intake can be found on Internet sites which promote anorexia. These "pro-ana" Web sites were developed for anorexics who want advice and support. For instance, one female wrote about her daily diet which consisted of a clementine, a cup of tea, one Special K® bar, one Lean Cuisine®, and a low-fat yogurt, for a total of about 350 calories. Another anorexic's daily intake consisted of two Special K® bars, 50 calories each of fruit and vegetables, for a total of 280 calories. Both also exercised throughout the day, trying to ensure that they burned more calories than they consumed ("The Anorexic Queen" 2008). Below, Ari describes her typical diet in detail:

> I ate one cup of Special K® cereal and I used a measuring cup to ensure that I did not eat any more calories than I had decided. For lunch, I ate an apple and a turkey sandwich that mostly consisted of two pieces of bread and a miniscule piece of turkey in-between. I would pull all of the crust off. At dinner, I ate one apple and a small piece of plain chicken. This totaled 400 calories, which I burned off easily by exercising two and a half hours per day. During meals, I would challenge myself not to eat the last bite of food, even though I was starving. Everything that I ate contained less than one hundred calories and the fat content was 1/6 the amount of the calories. I read every nutrition panel on boxes, even if I did not allow myself to eat the food.

When anorexics eat more than they had planned for a particular day, even by as little as ten calories, they often think they are failures and fear that they have gained a significant amount of weight. As a result, they punish themselves and go to extreme measures to increase their weight loss efforts. They may refrain from all food for a certain time period, begin a liquid diet, or make themselves vomit.

According to both classification systems, individuals with anorexia must also have a distorted body image or be unaware that their weight is truly as low as it is and far below the recommended IBW. Anorexics may look in the mirror and think that they are obese if they can see any breast tissue or can pinch the skin on their waist or hips. Or they may see excess skin hanging from their arms, legs, and buttocks, and interpret the skin as fat, rather than extra skin due to loss of fat and muscle. Many anorexics constantly compare themselves to others. They may hoard or cut out pictures of models and celebrities to try to look as thin as or thinner than their role models. They may look at other anorexics on pro-ana Web sites and think that they are fat compared to the anorexics in the photos. Their abnormal response to these images will be to increase their weight loss efforts. Ari remembers these distortions. "No matter how thin I was my stomach always bothered me. It was sunken in, yet I always saw it bulging with imaginary fat. All I focused on was diminishing the fat."

Another similarity between the classification systems is that they both require that females have amenorrhea to meet the criteria for anorexia. If teens have not yet begun puberty (prepubertal) or have not reached menarche, then they must have a delay in the onset of puberty or menarche. When someone has not yet begun puberty, it is much more difficult to make the diagnosis because the changes are more subtle. There may not be an actual weight loss but, instead, an insufficient amount of weight gain during a time when many peers are going through their growth spurts. This change on the growth curve can be missed by a physician or, alternatively, may be interpreted to mean that the preteen or teen simply hasn't started their pubertal growth spurt yet.

DIFFERENCES BETWEEN THE MAJOR MODELS USED TO DIAGNOSE ANOREXIA

Although most criteria used by the classification systems are similar, there are ways in which they differ. First of all, only the ICD-10 system specifically includes criteria for diagnosing anorexia in males. It includes behavioral changes, such as the loss of libido, which is often due to decreased levels of sex steroids in the body. The ICD-10 also notes that there can be a decrease in the levels of other hormones in either gender, such as growth hormone or thyroid hormone. The level of these hormones can drop when a body is in a starvation state and is trying to conserve energy. Also, whereas the DSM-IV-TR classifies two types of anorexia, depending on whether or not the person binges and/or purges, it doesn't require that someone exercise excessively or abuse medications to be diagnosed with anorexia, but the ICD-10 does. To meet the diagnosis of anorexia in the ICD-10 system, an individual must make themselves vomit, use appetite suppressants and/or diuretics, or exercise excessively for the purpose of losing weight. Those who do not exhibit one of these behaviors do not fulfill all the requirements for anorexia. Accordingly, in the ICD-10 system, individuals who meet all the criteria except the last would receive a diagnosis of "atypical anorexia nervosa." The American classification system does not have a similar diagnosis for individuals who meet all but one criterion.

WHAT HAPPENS WHEN SOMEONE DOESN'T MEET ALL THE CRITERIA

The DSM-IV-TR classifies people who have symptoms severe enough to have a significant eating disorder, but who do not meet all of the criteria for anorexia nervosa or other eating disorders, as having an eating disorder not otherwise specified (EDNOS). About 60% of eating disorder diagnoses fall into the EDNOS category (Striegel-Moore and Wonderlich 2007). Many experts think that this percentage is too high and that the criteria used to diagnose anorexia are too rigid. They believe that some people diagnosed with EDNOS actually have anorexia or a related disorder, bulimia. One reason individuals do not meet all the criteria for anorexia is that, although they are severely restricting their food intake, they were obese at the beginning of their illness and are not yet 15% below their IBW. Another reason some women are diagnosed with EDNOS rather than anorexia is because, despite meeting the other criteria for anorexia, they are still menstruating. Experts argue that whether or not females are menstruating has little to no impact on their eating disorder symptoms, thoughts, and long-term prognosis (Berkman, Lohr, and Bulik 2007). Furthermore, the use of an oral contraceptive pill or hormonal injection, which is common among females these days, can alter or totally inhibit menses irrespective of a female's actual weight.

Another example of individuals who do not meet all the criteria for anorexia is those who deny concerns about their weight or fear of becoming fat. This is particularly common in children and younger adolescents. In fact, it has been shown repeatedly that younger adolescents and individuals who don't want treatment sometimes deny that they have any fears regarding their weight. Also, children and preteens who diet or lose weight often aren't consciously aware or don't think that that they are afraid of becoming fat, even though their behaviors may indicate otherwise. In addition, they may not be able to understand or express their thoughts. Instead, some complain of a physical concern, such as a fear of choking, as a reason for their poor food intake. Consequently, some specialists have proposed that, instead of relying on a verbal admission of food fears, physicians observe or ask questions about behaviors which indicate a fear surrounding food and weight. This might include evidence that they are severely limiting their diet to only include foods such as lettuce and vegetables, refusing to attend functions which involve food, or purging regularly after meals.

Another reason for failing to meet all the criteria for anorexia is because, instead of losing weight, some individuals may simply not gain weight at a time when they should be going through their growth spurt and may have delayed puberty and menarche. To add to the confusion, some children may not have an eating disorder but, instead, are underweight because they are extremely picky eaters or because they misinterpreted advice given to them by a physician or nutritionist (Fisher 2006). All of these differences in the presentation between younger and older individuals makes experts question whether the diagnosis of EDNOS in young children and teens is similar to that seen in older adolescents and adults or whether they are, in fact, two distinct conditions. These are all important distinctions because the type of treatment, prognosis, and amount of reimbursement provided by private insurance companies all vary according to the diagnosis.

PSYCHIATRIC OR MEDICAL ILLNESS THAT MAY OCCUR ALONG WITH ANOREXIA

Many people who have anorexia nervosa have additional mental health issues or medical illnesses, called co-morbid diagnoses. In fact, studies have shown that as many as 80% of those with anorexia will have another psychiatric disorder at some point in their lives and over 70% will have a second disorder at the time they are diagnosed with anorexia. Two of the most common psychiatric illnesses that occur alongside anorexia are major depression and anxiety disorders. Depression tends to remain after the anorexia is treated. The likelihood that someone with anorexia will become depressed during their lifetime is 50% to 68% and the likelihood that they will suffer from anxiety is from 55% to 65% (Commission on Adolescent Eating Disorders 2007). Ari remembers her depression that coexisted with her anorexia. "I had deep depression during my anorexia nervosa. When I was in the company of others, I was morbid and my excuse was that I was exhausted. I cried incessantly and was always pessimistic. I had depression for months, even after my weight returned to normal."

Anxiety disorders frequently seen in people with anorexia include social phobias and obsessive-compulsive disorder; such individuals may acquire anxiety before they develop anorexia. Those with social phobias are afraid to be in a variety of situations where they must interact with others, while those who have obsessive-compulsive personality disorder are totally preoccupied with rules, orderliness, and control, or must repeat a task incessantly. Other common co-morbid diagnoses include substance abuse and personality disorders, such as dependent, avoidant, and passive-aggressive personality disorders. All interfere with normal living and can be disabling. In a dependent personality disorder, the affected person relies excessively on others and feels as if he is unable to cope or do anything on his own; he is very clingy. In an avoidant disorder, the person is very shy and feels inadequate. People who are passive-aggressive may appear to be compliant and in agreement about something with which they don't actually agree and then later or at other times can be openly angry and hostile, usually extreme for the given situation.

People with medical illnesses such as insulin-dependent diabetes, disorders of the stomach and intestines, and thyroid disease are also more likely to develop anorexia. Food and exercise are important components of these conditions, so those afflicted have to pay close attention to their nutritional and exercise habits. Certain foods should not be eaten because they can increase symptoms or cause serious, permanent medical complications. In addition, healthier, low-fat foods are generally better tolerated than foods high in fat and sugar. Furthermore, people with diabetes need to know that exercise and weight changes have a direct effect on their body's sugar level and the amount of insulin they need. Diabetics who exercise more or who weigh less often do not need as much insulin to maintain a normal glucose, or sugar level. Often, children with one of these illnesses will first visit their doctor because of weight loss, along with other symptoms. The combination of all these problems allows the doctor to make a diagnosis.

Sometimes the patient will consider the weight loss to be a positive aspect of the illness and will want to continue to lose weight. Even though they did not try to gain weight at first, they may begin to manipulate their medications to increase the loss. Diabetics who also have anorexia tend to lose weight by withholding or decreasing the dose of insulin they self-administer, which keeps the body from absorbing glucose into the bloodstream. Physicians may have a difficult time figuring out whether someone is losing weight because their diabetes is not under good control or because the patient is not taking the right dose of medicine. Anorexics with diabetes can lose a lot of weight by this method, but they can also cause permanent damage in their kidneys, nerves, blood vessels, and eyes—possibly leading to kidney failure, blindness, limb amputation, brain damage, and even death. People with gastrointestinal and thyroid disorders may also alter or stop taking their medications to lose weight. This also increases the possibility that they, too, will develop other severe medical complications. For example, those with an intestinal illness called inflammatory bowel disease may develop tears and adhesions in their intestines, suffer severe abdominal pain, become anemic, and develop nutritional deficiencies. Without appropriate treatment, they may need surgery to remove large parts of their intestine, sometimes emergently.

WARNING SIGNS

When parents notice several signs and symptoms that could be indicative of anorexia, they may bring their child to their physician to be evaluated. Alternatively, a physician may become concerned during a routine office visit that the patient has an eating disorder. The patient will be questioned, an exam will be performed, and the weight will be closely followed. There are many warning signs, when they occur together, that could point toward anorexia. These include:

- Dramatic weight loss
- Preoccupation with weight, food, calories, fat grams, and dieting
- Refusal to eat certain foods, progressing to restrictions against whole categories of food (e.g., no carbohydrates, etc.)
- Frequent comments about feeling "fat" or overweight despite weight loss
- Anxiety about gaining weight or being fat
- Denial of hunger
- Development of food rituals (e.g., eating foods in certain orders, excessive chewing, rearranging food on a plate)
- Consistent excuses to avoid mealtimes or situations involving food
- Excessive, rigid exercise regimen—despite weather, fatigue, illness, or injury—the need to "burn off" calories taken in
- Withdrawal from usual friends and activities
- Behaviors and attitudes indicating that weight loss, dieting and control of food are becoming primary concerns (Anorexia Nervosa and Related Eating Disorders, Inc. n.d.)

Initially, someone may only have a few of these signs or symptoms. When individuals, often teenagers, worry excessively about their weight or body size and shape, they may develop very rigid eating and exercise habits which can be so significant that they interfere with or change one's lifestyle. At this point, they have developed "disordered eating." They may begin to skip meals, develop secret eating rituals, and decide to lose a few pounds. They usually have a reason for deciding to lose weight. Perhaps they think it will make them look much better or that they will be more desirable to and accepted by others.

They may have disordered eating for months or years. On the other hand, these behaviors may increase in severity and they could develop anorexia nervosa.

MAKING A DIAGNOSIS OF ANOREXIA NERVOSA

Although anorexia nervosa is a common cause of weight loss in an otherwise healthy-appearing adolescent and young adult, it is not the only cause. In fact, even if patients admit that they are weight conscious and restrict their food intake, it does not automatically mean that they have anorexia. One of the first and most important things a physician must do is make sure that someone who has lost weight does not have a medical or psychiatric condition rather than, or in addition to anorexia (see Table 3.1). Therefore, a physician must obtain a thorough clinical history from the patient and the patient's family and perform a complete physical. Questions or concerns that come up during the history or physical will lead the doctor toward specific laboratory tests or special studies which might help identify a condition.

Table 3.1
Differential Diagnosis of Anorexia Nervosa

Medical Pathology
Gastrointestinal:
  Inflammatory bowel disease, celiac, and other malabsorption syndromes; achalasia, superior mesenteric artery syndrome
Endocrine:
  Hyperthyroidism, diabetes mellitus type 1, Addison disease, hypothalamic tumors, Sheehan syndrome
  Emaciating diseases:
  AIDS, tuberculosis, metastatic cancers, cystic fibrosis
Obstetric:
  Hyperemesis gravidarum

Behavioral/Psychiatric Pathology
Developmental variation:
  Dieting/body image variation, dieting body image problems
Other eating disorders:
  Eating disorder, not otherwise specified, bulimia nervosa, food avoidance emotional disorder, selective eating, functional dysphagia, pervasive refusal syndrome
Other psychiatric disorders:
  Major depression, psychosis/schizophrenia, substance abuse (cocaine, amphetamines), social phobia, obsessive compulsive disorder, dysmorphophobia

There are several systems within the body which, when they aren't functioning properly, can cause medical illnesses along with significant weight loss. These include problems with the stomach and intestines (the gastrointestinal tract), the endocrine system, and complications due to pregnancy. In addition, illnesses such as cancer and lupus, which affect many organs in the body, are frequently accompanied by weight loss. Sometimes, gastrointestinal diseases, including inflammatory bowel and celiac disease, can be mistaken for anorexia in an adolescent. Inflammatory bowel disease is an irritation of the intestines, and celiac disease is a sensitivity to products containing gluten, which includes wheat and other grains. People with these illnesses often limit their food intake and have significant weight loss because they realize that eating certain types of foods increases pain and diarrhea. In addition to weight loss, they may have delayed puberty and poor nutrition, other problems also noted in people with anorexia. A helpful clue during the interview which points toward a gastrointestinal disease is a history of diarrhea, especially when accompanied by blood or mucus, and abdominal pain. Other problems that can occur with inflammatory bowel disease include arthritis and skin rashes.

Laboratory tests can also help determine whether someone is more likely to have anorexia or another medical condition. When a patient has significant weight loss, tests that would point toward a medical reason include an elevated sedimentation which indicates general irritation within the body, anemia due to blood loss, and low protein levels because of severe malnutrition. If a physician is concerned about a gastrointestinal problem, then an endoscopy, a procedure where a scope is used to look directly at the intestines or esophagus, may be helpful. If necessary, a small piece of tissue can be removed and analyzed. There are also less common gastrointestinal conditions that can lead to weight loss. For example, some people feel as if they are choking while they swallow, which may lead to vomiting after meals. People with these uncomfortable sensations often don't eat much and, therefore, lose weight. Special radiological procedures, such as a barium swallow or an upper gastrointestinal series with small bowel follow through can be performed to look for this problem, in addition to others (Fisher 2006).

ANOREXIA MUST BE DIFFERENTIATED FROM ENDOCRINE DISORDERS

Other medical conditions, such as endocrine disorders, which cause abnormal hormone levels in the body, can lead to significant weight loss, in addition to amenorrhea in females. For example, one hormone abnormality which causes impressive, rapid weight loss is Graves' disease, a condition where the body attacks its own thyroid gland and causes it to make too much thyroid hormone. Unlike anorexia, however, people with Graves' disease often have a characteristic wide-eyed, wild look to their eyes called "exophthalmos." They also have an enlarged thyroid gland which can be felt in the front of the neck, a very fast heart rate, and a high blood pressure. In addition, they constantly complain of being hungry and eat often. Their thyroid levels will be abnormally high and will confirm the diagnosis. Another example is insulin-dependent diabetes, where patients not only have rapid weight loss, but because they also complain of being thirsty and drinking all the time, they urinate much more often and become dehydrated. In addition, diseases of an organ in the brain called the hypothalamus can cause not only weight loss, but also changes in the heart rate, blood pressure, and body temperature, as well as complaints of headaches and vision problems. Conditions which involve other organs that produce hormones, such as the pituitary gland in the brain and the adrenal gland in the abdomen, can also cause weight loss but have other signs and symptoms that are not characteristic of anorexia (Treasure, Schmidt, and Van Furth 2003).

WEIGHT LOSS CAN BE THE FIRST SIGN OF A SYSTEMIC ILLNESS

There are also many systemic illnesses—those that involve the entire body—which can lead to weight loss, and sometimes it is the first sign of an illness. This can happen with diseases such as cancer, cystic fibrosis, tuberculosis, as well as autoimmune and immunologic disorders such as AIDS. Through questioning, the physician may find clues that the weight loss is due to something other than anorexia. For example, the patient may admit to having multiple sexual partners, recurrent or prolonged fevers, a frequent cough, or severe or recurrent infections. When a physician examines the patient, there may be abnormalities in the lungs, liver, spleen, or lymph nodes which would indicate a different type of medical problem. Often the laboratory workup and special tests such as a skin test for tuberculosis (PPD), genetic testing or a special procedure (sweat test) for cystic fibrosis, a complete blood count and measurements of liver and kidney function for cancer, or an evaluation of immune function for AIDS will lead to a diagnosis. One final medical condition which deserves mentioning is hypergravidum of pregnancy. Sometimes pregnant women have severe and prolonged morning sickness, which makes them vomit so much that they can't keep any food down and end up losing weight. A teen in this predicament might be afraid to tell anybody that she is pregnant, so she keeps her vomiting a secret. A simple history and pregnancy test will confirm this diagnosis.

PSYCHIATRIC CONDITIONS CAN CAUSE WEIGHT LOSS

Various psychiatric conditions can also lead to weight loss. Although depression can occur alongside anorexia, sometimes people who just have major depression can lose their appetite or desire to eat. It can be difficult to decipher which came first—the lack of a desire to eat or the depression. Schizophrenia can also lead to or even present with weight loss if the ill person has hallucinations or delusions. For example, he might think that someone is trying to poison him so he refuses to eat. Or he may hear voices telling him to stop eating every time he sits down for a meal. In addition, phobias and personality disorders can also lead to weight loss. For example, someone may not want to eat in front of others because of a fear or feeling of inadequacy. A person with compulsive or obsessive eating behaviors may be limited in the amount they can eat at one sitting because they feel they have to chew each bite fifty times or wipe their mouth repeatedly after each forkful of food. Drug abuse can decrease the desire to eat. Drugs such as cocaine act as an appetite suppressant. Additionally, if someone is addicted to a drug, most of the time and money may be spent looking for that particular drug and getting high, rather than thinking about the next meal.

Some people, mostly children and teens, have problems with food for reasons that are not related at all to their weight or a fear of becoming fat. For example, some children are very picky or selective eaters. On physical exam and history, however, their weight is usually normal and they don't have issues regarding body shape. Other children may have a condition known as functional dysphagia, where they feel as if they are choking when they swallow food or liquids. They tend not to eat too much because they hate the feeling that occurs with it.

TAKING A COMPLETE HISTORY—THE FIRST STEP
IN DIAGNOSING ANOREXIA NERVOSA

Optimally, the answers that an anorexic and family provide to questions during an interview will make the diagnosis of anorexia likely so that the physical exam and laboratory tests will serve mainly to confirm the doctor's suspicions. However, patients are often in denial or unreliable due to their age or because they want to be secretive about their weight loss and behaviors. Ari insisted that her limited food intake was for good reasons. "I was aiming to be number one on the varsity tennis team and I had to work hard to reach that goal. I promised that I would increase my caloric intake, but I just agreed with anything that allowed my anorexic habits to persist." There are many screening instruments available, such as the *Clinical Eating Disorder Rating*

Instrument, the *Eating Disorder Examination*, the *Interview for Diagnosis of Eating Disorders*, the *Structured Interview for Anorexia and Bulimia Nervosa*, and the *Eating Attitudes Test* that can help a physician gather important information during the visit (Levey n.d.).

Self-completed questionnaires and symptom checklists can also be helpful. If the patient is forthcoming, she may discuss a fear of becoming fat and will recall her very limited food and caloric intake. This information, combined with a weight which is very low for the age and height, should alert the physician to the possibility of anorexia. If, however, she refuses to answer questions or denies any changes in her eating habits, her family may be able to provide some answers. Sometimes, however, the family isn't aware of the limited food intake or distorted body image. Occasionally, they are also in denial and are unable to see that their child has an eating and weight loss problem. Anorexics can do a very good job of hiding their fears and true daily intake from their families and friends for quite a while. Tactics used to secretly avoid eating food include cutting it into small pieces on plates, piling it in ways that make it look like the majority has been eaten, hiding it in napkins to throw away later, and self-inducing vomiting after dinner. Ari recalls tactics some anorexics used to hide their weight loss such as putting change in their pockets or drinking several bottles of water right before weigh-ins.

Since anorexics are known to be secretive and manipulative with regard to their weight loss and food intake, they may or may not admit the use or, more appropriately, abuse of laxatives and diuretics. They are more likely to discuss their exercise regimen, which is often rather excessive. They may exercise for several hours a day or even several times daily. Sometimes a parent will comment that they hear their child doing jumping jacks or crunches in the bedroom at all hours of the day and night. Ari recalls her exercise regimen during the height of her anorexia.

> *Every single day I ran five miles, did 100 crunches, and shook my legs. I even continued my runs in the pouring rain. I literally sprinted to the parking lot after school so that I could get home quickly and start exercising again. When I returned home from school, my second exercise regimen of the day progressed. I had to play tennis for at least an hour and a half to feel good. My feet were not allowed to stop moving for a moment and I ran in place between points and sprinted to retrieve tennis balls. On stairs and in school hallways, I would sprint up all of them. When I studied, I paced my room for hours. When I sat down, I would lay my head off of the chair so that my abs were stretched and my legs had to support me; I stayed like this for long periods of time with the blood rushing to my head. I took advantage of every opportunity to exercise no matter how silly I appeared. Each day I ensured that I burned*

*more calories than I took in. I constantly calculated everything I ate compared
to my activities. I was obsessive enough to calculate driving to school, shaking
my legs, and even showering.*

Although the patient may or may not actually admit to fears surrounding their
weight and shape of their body, a helpful clue is the denial of any other problems
that tend to be associated with other medical illnesses. However, it is important
to know that young teens and children are more likely to try to relate medical
symptoms to their weight loss than are older adolescents and adults. The physician must be aware that some complaints which actually are due to a medical
problem are as a result of complications from anorexia. For example, chest pain
and upper abdominal tenderness can be caused by esophagitis or an esophageal
tear (called a Mallory-Weiss tear) due to purging or self-induced vomiting.

PERFORMING A COMPLETE PHYSICAL EXAMINATION
IS ESSENTIAL

Sometimes, during our daily routines, we will pass by someone who is
extremely thin. If they don't appear ill in any other way, many of us will
assume they have anorexia. Other times, however, we will pass by someone
who looks thin, but not excessively. We might wish we were as thin as they or,
alternatively, we may not even notice them. The characteristic features of anorexics will be easily noticed at times, but not always, especially when they first
become ill. When patients first visit a doctor for a weight loss evaluation, or
even for an entirely different problem altogether, the physician may notice that
they look rather thin but they may not have other obvious features of anorexia.
However, with time and further weight loss they begin to look skeletal with
typically drawn faces and sunken cheekbones due to a lack of fat. Their bones
become easily visualized, particularly their hip bones and shoulder blades,
which protrude much more than usual. Their legs and arms have no visible fat
on them. Their hands and feet become particularly pale and blue, or acrocya-
notic. Their skin hangs down, making them look much older than their actual
age. They wear heavy clothes, not only to hide their body, but also because
they are always cold. Their weight, by definition, will be at least 15% below
that which is ideal for the height and age, and frequently much lower.

Other aspects of an examination aren't as readily apparent and require careful measurements and evaluation. If the patient is young, the physician may
notice that puberty is delayed. If the body is in a starvation state, the metabolism will decrease, and the physician will notice a low body temperature, heart
rate, and blood pressure. The doctor may order blood pressures in different
positions to document whether there is any orthostatic hypotension (a drop in

blood pressure when someone sits or stands from a lying position). This can occur in anorexics who are dehydrated. Ari remembers the consequences of a low body temperature and lack of fat on her body. "I endlessly shook and had goose bumps all over my body. I could never warm up, no matter how long I stood in hot showers or in front of fires. My bones ached from the cold. Every day I wore four layers of shirts and sweatshirts to keep warm and give me an appearance of body fat."

The physician may also notice the acrocyanosis, which can occur when the body decreases blood flow to the extremities to try to conserve energy. The appearance of the skin, hair, and nails will also change. Skin may become dry and yellow, which can be partly explained by an increased consumption of orange vegetables, such as carrots, but researchers don't think this completely explains the change in skin color. Fine hair, or lanugo, will grow on the body, and scalp hair will become thin or begin to fall out. Nails will become brittle and will break easily. On an exam of muscle strength, there will be an overall generalized sense of weakness. It is possible that there will be signs of multiple organ failure, including heart, kidney, or liver; swelling of the extremities; a bloated abdomen; an irregularity in pulse; shortness of breath; and/or fluid in the lungs. The physician may also notice that the patient has slow, monotonous speech and a difficult time focusing. This could be indicative of organic brain syndrome, another complication of anorexia. In retrospect, Ari remembers the problems she had while trying to study during high school. "I had intense problems focusing on my studies; work that at one time took me an hour, would take me three hours to complete to my level of perfection. I did not do well on my SATs because I had a lot of trouble focusing after the second section. Even a fifty minute test drained me of all my energy." During the physical, the physician will also look for evidence that the patient has been purging. For example, there may be cavities and a loss of enamel on the teeth due to acids in the vomited food particles that pass by the teeth. Other signs include chipped teeth due to forceful purging, swollen parotid glands in the back of the cheeks, and calluses on the back of the hands (Russell's Sign), indicating that fingers are being used to induce vomiting.

Laboratory Tests and Special Procedures May Be Needed to Diagnose Anorexia

All newly diagnosed anorexics should have laboratory tests done to make sure there isn't another medical problem that is being missed and to provide further support for the diagnosis (See Table 3.2). There are several normal and abnormal lab values which are characteristic of anorexia. On the standard

Table 3.2
Laboratory Evaluation

Test	Results
Complete blood cell count*	Hemoconcentration, leukopenia, thrombocytopenia
ESR*	Increase suggests another illness
Clinical chemistry*	Reduced blood sugar, calcium, magnesium, phosphate; reduced urea, electrolyte abnormalities; abnormal LFTs, elevated amylase
Nutritional parameters*	Prealbumin, transferrin: low with fasting; total protein, normal. Low albumin may imply another disease. Cholesterol often high
Urine analysis*	High specific gravity in dehydration; low in isosthenuria and water intoxication. Proteinuria, hematuria with exercise. Blue urine: diuretic abuse
Pregnancy test*	Confirms absence of pregnancy as the cause of amenorrhea
TSH, T3	T3 low in the presence of normal TSH— Malnutrition
Sex hormones	Confirm hypothalamic hypogonadism—low estradiol
Serum osmolality	Decreased in water loading, NaQ 120 mEq/L: risk for seizures
Investigation for celiac disease or IBD, endoscopies	If GI disease is suspected
Vitamin levels, zinc	Pernicious anemia, scurvy, pellagra, acrodermatitis, carotene
ECG	Bradycardia, hypokalemia, arrhythmia, prolonged QT interval
Urine drug tests	Amphetamines
Neuroimaging	Brain atrophy, loss of white and gray matter; if headaches, to evaluate for CNS tumor
Pelvic ultrasound	To detect follicular development
Bone density by dexa scan	Osteopenia/osteoporosis with more than 6 months of amenorrhea
Research tests	Genetic markers, bone metabolites, functional MRI, leptin, Grehlin

*Routine tests.
Abbreviations: CNS, central nervous system; ECG, electrocardiogram; ESR, Erythrocyte sedimentation rate; GI, gastrointestinal; IBD, inflammatory bowel disease; LFTs, liver function tests; MRI, magnetic resonance imaging; Na, sodium; TSH, thyrotropin; T3, triiodothyronine.
Source: Reprinted from *Advances in Pediatrics*, Vol. 52, Tomas Silber, "Anorexia Nervosa Among Children and Adolescents" Pgs.49-76, Copyright © 2005, with permission from Elsevier.

blood tests a *complete blood count* may show slight anemia due to nutritional deficiency and a slightly low white blood count. The *erythrocyte sedimentation rate* (ESR), a generalized measure of inflammation in the body, should be normal and, if not, would suggest that there might be another medical illness affecting multiple systems. The *metabolic profile*, which includes a measure of the concentration or levels of salts, magnesium, phosphate, proteins, and kidney and liver function in the blood could show many abnormalities for a variety of reasons. The physician must evaluate all the possibilities to decide which seems most reasonable. For example, overloading on water, abusing laxatives or diuretics, and purging can all cause electrolyte abnormalities which will be picked up on the lab tests. When an anorexic drinks a lot of water to feel full or to increase the weight before a "weigh in," the concentration of sodium (hyponatremia) in the body could decrease to dangerously low levels. Similarly, self-inducted vomiting could rid the body of potassium and chloride. Abuse of diuretics or laxatives can also lead to low levels of potassium (hypokalemia) but high levels of sodium and chloride due to dehydration and diarrhea. Other blood tests which may be abnormal in anorexics include glucose, magnesium, phosphate, and cholesterol. In addition, when a physician is evaluating someone with potential anorexia, close attention will be paid to liver and kidney function tests to make sure that there is absolutely no evidence of organ failure as a result of chronic starvation, malnutrition, or medication abuse.

Next, a sample of urine must be tested, called a *urinalysis*, which may show a high specific gravity, which indicates dehydration. The urine test may also show evidence that protein and blood are being spilled into the urine, which can occur with excessive exercise. To be complete, a physician should also order both a *pregnancy test* in all females, even young adolescents, to ensure that pregnancy isn't the cause of amenorrhea, and *thyroid function tests* to assess for a general dysfunction of the hypothalamus in the brain. An *estradiol level* in females, and a *testosterone level* in males, might also be performed for similar reasons. Finally, an electrocardiogram (ECG) needs to be done to make sure that purging or medication abuse hasn't caused problems with the heart such as disturbance of the heart rhythm, known as an arrhythmia or a prolonged QT interval, which is a type of disturbance of the conduction system of the heart. It will also help detect an enlarged heart or other cardiac abnormalities resulting from chronic starvation and, therefore, should be done even if the patient denies purging or abusing medications.

If a patient is more than 15% below the ideal body weight (IBW), several additional studies should be done to rule out other possible problems. For one thing, the heart may be enlarged, which can immediately be noted on a chest radiograph (CXR). In addition, uric acid levels should be checked to look for high levels in those who abuse laxatives. Also, a special urine collection, called a 24 hour creatinine clearance, should be performed to evaluate kidney function. Bone loss is a very common problem that occurs in anorexics who remain at least 15% below their IBW for six months or longer. For this reason, a Dual Energy X-Ray Absorptiometry (DEXA scan) is performed to search for decreased bone mass. Physicians are also aware that anorexics who are 20% or more below their IBW are at risk of developing problems with their ability to think and reason. If they have evidence of neurologic problems, a brain scan should be done to evaluate for organic brain syndrome. Lastly, those who are 30% or more below that expected for their age should have special skin testing to look for problems with immune function, which is the body's ability to fight off infections.

Weight loss is seen in many chronic illnesses, and is not just a symptom of anorexia nervosa. There are strict criteria which someone must meet to be diagnosed with anorexia. Sometimes, blood tests and other special procedures are performed, especially if the physician is unclear regarding the diagnosis. In addition, specific tests may also be ordered if a physician is concerned about specific complications due to anorexia.

4

Characteristics of Those Who Develop Anorexia

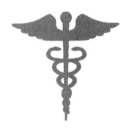

"Before I was diagnosed with anorexia nervosa, I appeared to be the perfect overachiever from the outside."

—Ari

THE TYPE OF PERSON WHO DEVELOPS ANOREXIA NERVOSA

There has been a significant increase in the incidence and prevalence of anorexia nervosa in recent years. This has led to greater interest in the illness and, consequently, more studies have been conducted which have provided us with a better understanding of this topic. Through statistical analyses, researchers have determined that about 1% of females in the United States are diagnosed with anorexia, and approximately 6% of all anorexics are males. Researchers have also determined that, in general, those with a particular set of personality features are more likely to develop anorexia nervosa than others. In addition, there are several risk factors which may predispose someone to developing the illness. For instance, we have known that, even as far back as the 1800s, girls are much more likely to develop anorexia than boys. Through historical accounts and more recent statistical analyses, we have also learned that most girls who develop anorexia are teens and young adults, although older women are certainly not immune. In relatively recent years, it has been documented that specific ethnic groups in the United States are more likely to be diagnosed with anorexia than others, with Caucasians being at greatest risk (Chao et al. 2008).

For years it was thought that anorexia was an illness seen exclusively in Caucasian girls from the middle- or upper-socioeconomic classes, or from fairly successful Caucasian families who were high achievers moving up socially and economically. The typical at-risk girls were described as attractive and privileged, who were given "everything," including a good education, nice clothing, a variety of food choices, shelter above and beyond the necessary, and many opportunities. One or both parents were often very attentive and extremely involved in their upbringing. Clinicians thought that fathers, in particular, expected their children to excel not just in academics, but also in other areas of life, such as sports and leadership qualities. New research has demonstrated that, although these characteristics may contribute to the development of anorexia, they are not the sole cause.

Some experts believe that children brought up in this type of environment may think they don't deserve anything they are given and, therefore, try to earn these lavish extras by always pleasing their parents. As a result, they act and behave differently than they normally would. By living their lives according to others' desires and by spending most of their time and energy wondering what others want, they never discover their own needs or desires. Outwardly, they appear to be ideal children because they never complain or cause problems. Their parents are proud of them; the children perform exactly as the parents want. The children are very successful at it; inwardly, however, they always feel inadequate, as if they are never doing a good enough job. Their persistent feelings of inadequacy and lack of development of their own persona may predispose them to developing anorexia (Levenkron 2000).

In the mid-1970s, several personality features were identified that appear to be common in those who develop anorexia. Reportedly, these (mostly) girls are likely to be perfectionists who have obsessive and compulsive personalities. They are often described as respectful, cooperative, and nonconfrontational. They may strive for straight As in school or practice a particular sport for hours on end so that they can prove they are the best player on the team. They may stay awake half the night studying for a quiz or do the majority of the work in a group assignment. This perfectionism also carries over into social situations, where they are often very outgoing and have a charming personality. Ari recalls her junior year of high school, when she took five honors and advanced placement classes, striving not only to get straight As, but also the highest As in each class. To do this, she remained awake until 1 a.m. most school days, memorizing her facts forward and backward. She was also ranked first on her tennis team and spent hours each day trying to improve her strokes and exercise tolerance.

Underneath their facade, however, these individuals are often inhibited and anxious, and don't like to express or share their true feelings with others (Pryor and Wiederman 1998). Specialists think that many of them, for a variety of reasons, don't develop a healthy, trusting dependence with either of their parents and, consequently, try to reassure themselves when they are distressed rather than reach out to others. Because they think that they can't turn to or depend on others, they may develop a feeling of "emptiness," a negative self-esteem, and a poor self-identity. Some theorists think that, as part of a poor self-identity, females fail to develop a sense of femininity. Until these individuals develop anorexia, they can often successfully hide their feelings of inadequacy by working hard to become successful in many areas of life, including academic, athletic, and social arenas. In describing her own life before anorexia, Ari writes, "I always believed that I was setting the perfect example for my siblings, and my parents praised me for being an amazing daughter and role model. I was the girl defined as super sweet and innocent. The truth is, I was a pushover who thrived on pleasing others and I did not have my own identity."

THE POSSIBLE PARENTAL CONTRIBUTION TO ANOREXIA

In addition to describing a particular type of person who is more likely to develop anorexia, several years ago therapists suggested that there is a specific type of family and family-child interaction which predisposes a child to developing anorexia. They portray a mother who is very involved, sometimes too much, in her child's life, making many decisions for her child. While the mothers appear to be secure and self-assured, many worry about their own appearance and may spend a lot of time talking about dieting and weight problems, even if they aren't overweight. Some have had or continue to have eating disorders. They often look at women's magazines, comparing themselves to models in the advertisements. Fathers, on the other hand, may have a different role in the lives of their children. At times they, too, may also be over-involved, pushing their child to excel in many areas of life. Other times, however, therapists note an obvious void in their daughters' lives for many reasons, including long work hours, a chronic medical or mental illness, divorce, death, or even the lack of desire to become involved (Levenkron 2000). Both parents tend to be well-educated and successful. They expect their child to conform to their own ideals and may dictate what their child should take interest in and how she (or he) should behave, perhaps never listening to or approving of her side of a disagreement. The parents are proud of their "perfect" family and speak positively about their home environment. There seems to be an overall sense of conformity, where negative feelings or actions are not discussed or seen.

ETHNICITY, CULTURE, AND THE DEVELOPMENT OF ANOREXIA

Between 1987 and 2001, a large review and analysis was done on 18 studies to determine the role ethnicity and culture played on the development of anorexia. The results demonstrated that, while Caucasian females are more likely to develop anorexia than any other ethnic group, it does exist in a variety of ethnic and socioeconomic settings (Franko et al. 2007). After Caucasians, the group at greatest risk of developing anorexia is Asians, followed by Hispanics, and then African Americans (Chao et al. 2008). These ethnic variations may be due, in part, to cultural differences in the way women perceive themselves and their bodies, as demonstrated by research done with African American women. Based on surveys conducted between 1995 and 2005, African American women continue to be less likely to go on diets and are more satisfied and comfortable with their bodies than other ethnic groups. Studies have also shown that African American women are less likely than Caucasians to base their self-esteem on their physical appearance or to feel pressured to be thin, even at a young age. A survey conducted on elementary school children between third and sixth grades found that, in general, African American girls didn't relate physical appearance to weight, while Caucasian girls did. Additionally, African American men prefer women who are significantly larger than those preferred by Caucasian men (Lawrence and Thelen 1995). It is possible that all of these cultural differences contribute to a decreased risk of developing anorexia in the African American population.

Over the years, studies have indicated that there are differences in the prevalence of anorexia not only among various ethnicities within the United States, but also throughout different regions of the world, and that these variations appear to be based on a particular society's cultural views and socioeconomic status. Until recently, anorexia was found mainly in the industrialized regions of the world, such as the United States, Canada, and Western Europe, but was extremely rare or nonexistent in poorer, non-Westernized countries. One theory as to why anorexia didn't exist in the latter societies is because those who starve themselves in a poor country are unable to differentiate themselves from others, do not feel unique, and cannot make a personal or psychological statement through self-starvation. Consequently, self-starvation does not lead to greater control and satisfaction. This is one theory as to why the incidence of eating disorders decreases during economically difficult times, such as in Italy during World War II (Selvini-Palozzoli 1985).

HOW WESTERNIZATION INFLUENCES THE DEVELOPMENT OF ANOREXIA

More recently, researchers have found that the incidence of anorexia and eating disordered behaviors has increased in countries where it was previously rare or even nonexistent. While this increase may be due to improved diagnosis and more careful observation, it is also possible that this is a new phenomenon due to the Westernization of these other societies. For example, the increase in the number of people diagnosed with anorexia in Japan coincided with the end of World War II, when Western influence was first introduced. Additionally, other countries that have had a relatively recent influx of Western ideas and values, such as India, Egypt, Hong Kong, and Africa, are now also finding cases of anorexia and disordered eating for the first time (Nasser 1997). The possible impact of Western values on the introduction of or increase in anorexia in other countries is clearly seen by an event which occurred on the island of Fiji in the 1990s. Traditionally, their culture emphasizes robust and plump women and discourages dieting and exercise. Until the 1990s, they had reported only one case of anorexia. In 1995, Western customs were introduced when television was brought onto the island, along with TV programs depicting Western society. Researchers on Fiji surveyed school girls one month and three years after television was introduced. They found that prolonged exposure to television was associated with a significantly greater number of girls who exhibited disordered eating behaviors and who made themselves vomit to lose weight. The researchers also documented changing attitudes regarding diet, weight loss, and superficial appearance in the school girls, despite the fact that their parents wanted them to follow traditional customs of their own culture. Many school girls made comments about the television shows which indicated their desire to be thin and emulate the actresses on TV. For example, one girl said, "When I look at the characters on TV, the way they act on TV and I just look at the body, the figure of that body, so I say, 'look at them, they are thin and they all have this figure,' so I myself want to become like that, to become thin" (Becker et al. 2002).

Other countries have also looked into factors that increase the risk of developing anorexia in their populations. A study done in 2003 in Sweden, where it is possible to evaluate the entire population, demonstrated that many of their risk factors are similar to those seen in the United States. Although the average age of onset of anorexia is older in Sweden, 17 years versus 14 years of age, risk factors that were similar included gender, ethnicity, socioeconomic status, and psychosocial issues. Similar to the United States, teens in Sweden who had complications surrounding their own birth, such as anemia or neurologic problems, were at an increased risk of developing anorexia. Both countries also found that a child who had a parent with a psychiatric disorder, who had been in foster care, or who had been adopted from another country had a greater risk of developing anorexia. In addition, males in both the United States and in Sweden who developed anorexia were more likely to be overweight at the start of their illness than females. They were also more likely to be from a lower socioeconomic class. There also appears to be a cultural component to the development of anorexia. People who lived in Sweden but were originally from a country at lower risk of developing anorexia were more likely to develop anorexia than others from their native country (Lindberg and Hjern 2003). Other Westernized countries have also found that people who move there from other countries tend to have a greater risk of developing anorexia than they would if they remained in their native country.

ANOREXIA NERVOSA IN MALES

Although anorexia occurs mostly in females, it can also occur in males and studies show that the numbers are increasing. There have been several historical descriptions of adolescent boys in the seventeenth through nineteenth centuries who refused to eat but were healthy otherwise. Many historians assume that these males had anorexia, yet it had not been well-defined in this gender until recently. This may be because males don't fit all the criteria required to diagnose anorexia, such as the criterion requiring the loss of periods. Or, perhaps it is because the incidence of anorexia in men is so much lower than in women that the emphasis has been placed on females, while studies involving males have been largely ignored. However, there has been a relatively recent increase in awareness of anorexia in general, and the media over the past several years in particular has focused more on men's bodies and physical appearance. Consequently, anorexic males are being described and studied more over the past 10 to 20 years than previously.

FEATURES OF ANOREXIA THAT DIFFER BETWEEN MALES AND FEMALES

There are several aspects of anorexia that differ between males and females. To begin, its onset is later in males, with the typical age range being between

18 and 26 years of age rather than 15 to 18 years, which is typical for females. The later age of onset seen in boys may occur because they go through puberty about two years after girls, a common time for anorexia to develop. Alternatively, it may be because it is recognized later in males than in females, possibly because physicians are not looking for it. Another difference between the genders is that males don't have the same obsession with weight but, instead, focus more on muscle development. Males are more likely to exercise excessively and less likely to abuse laxatives or diet pills (Braun 1997). Yet, like females, about half of males will binge and purge. Third, they don't develop amenorrhea, an objective measure of significant weight loss in females. In addition, males often go to greater measures to hide the fact that they have a "female's illness" because it can be embarrassing for them. Importantly, males may be more likely to have a concomitant personality disorder than females, such as dependent, avoidant, and passive-aggressive personalities. All of these disorders interfere with normal living and can be disabling In addition, males are more likely to have a personal and family history of substance abuse (Treasure, Schmidt, and Van Furth 2003).

Whereas many females who diet and develop anorexia are not overweight before they develop anorexia, this is not true with males. Males are much more likely to be obese when they first begin their weight loss efforts, and they often report that they were teased about their weight. A college survey done several years ago found that women are much more likely than men to inaccurately label themselves as overweight. Forty-eight percent of randomly-selected women who completed a questionnaire thought that they were fat, compared to 26% of the men. A study done in 1987 documented that high school girls were four times more likely than boys to be trying to lose weight at the time of the study, while the boys were three times more likely to be trying to gain weight. In the study, males used exercise more often than women as a method of weight control. The males were also more likely to be satisfied with their weight, in general, and felt good about their bodies if they exercised regularly. Studies from the early 1990s supported previous trends. In a random survey conducted on over 11,000 high school students, 44% of females and 15% of males were trying to lose weight at the time of the survey (Serdula et al. 1993). Although females continue to be much more concerned about their weight and dieting, the gap between the percentage of men and women who diet is decreasing. In addition, a study published in 2006 showed that males are becoming more dissatisfied with their bodies. A recent random survey conducted on 14- to 16-year-old boys found that, while they said that they were satisfied with their appearance, some divulged that they more concerned with their appearance than they were willing to admit (Hargreaves and Tiggemann 2006).

THE RELATIONSHIP BETWEEN SEXUALITY
AND ANOREXIA IN MALES

Sexuality appears to be related to anorexia nervosa in males. Homosexuality, asexuality, and sexual anxieties have all been associated with anorexia in males. One study conducted on male anorexics found that 80% grew up in a home where sex was a taboo subject. Other research has shown that males who lose weight actually feel a sense of relief when they lose their sex drive, a phenomenon that occurs when their testosterone levels decrease. More specifically, 95% of anorexic males surveyed were relieved by the lack of libido that accompanied their weight loss and, furthermore had been trying to control their sex drive even before they developed anorexia. Additional support for a connection between sexual conflicts and anorexia is given by results of a survey, which determined that both homosexual and heterosexual anorexics felt anxious about their own sexuality, and 75% felt disgust regarding sexual relationships (Treasure, Schmidt, and Van Furth 2003). Also, males with anorexia are much less likely than females to have had any sexual relationships before the onset of their illness.

Males with anorexia tend to have more feminine attributes than their counterparts. They score high on the "femininity" aspect of personality profiles and view themselves as more feminine, both in terms of attitude and behavior. They also report feeling closer to their mothers than their fathers. In addition, male homosexuals are overrepresented in many studies of anorexia. While they represent approximately 5% of the male population in the United States, they comprise up to 42% of all males with eating disorders (Anorexia Nervosa and Related Eating Disorders, Inc. n.d.). Researchers have postulated that there is a "homosexual conflict" which may precede the onset of an eating disorder in up to one-half of male patients. Boys who are conflicted and anxious about their sexuality, particularly if they find themselves attracted to other males, may lose weight in an attempt to decrease or totally eliminate their libido and, subsequently, control their internal anxieties. Additionally, losing weight may decrease their attractiveness toward others and bring their bodies closer toward their prepubertal state. Alternatively, those who have accepted their homosexuality are aware of the greater emphasis this culture places on being thin and, in fact, this group of males is more likely to diet to lose weight. A study done in 1990 found that homosexual men are significantly thinner than heterosexual men. Homosexual men have reported feeling less satisfied with their bodies than heterosexuals, and find that their self-esteem and positive self-identity is more dependent on their appearance and overall weight than it is in heterosexuals.

Once males have passed through the initial stages of weight loss and have met the criteria for anorexia, their signs and symptoms become quite similar to those seen in females. They, too, become preoccupied with dieting and food, weigh themselves frequently, develop food rituals, have a distorted body image, and are compulsive with regard to exercise. As seen in women with anorexia, men also isolate themselves socially, have a strong need to be in control, develop rigid and inflexible thinking, and have a low self-esteem. Physically, the changes that occur in their bodies basically mirror those seen in females. Obviously, one major difference is that, instead of having a decrease in estrogen levels, they have a drop in testosterone levels, the main sex hormone seen in males.

LORI'S STORY: THE DEVELOPMENT OF ANOREXIA

Lori Gottlieb wrote *Stick Figure: A Diary of My Former Self*, based on a diary she kept over a one-year period, during which time she developed anorexia nervosa. Her story provides details about herself and her interactions with her family.

In the beginning of the book, at age 11 years, she writes about how she thinks she looks fine and that she enjoys eating a variety of foods. Her mother and her friends' mothers, on the other hand, talk incessantly about dieting and losing weight so they can look good and sexy. They are into fashion and physical appearance. Lori's mom tries to influence her daughter by pestering her to dress better—or "sexier," use makeup, and eat less so that she can "attract a man." Although Lori isn't overweight, her mom constantly talks to her about avoiding sweets so she can maintain a good figure. Even when they bake homemade cookies together, her mother makes Lori save them for her brother and dad, the men in the family. Her mom also stresses that a woman must always leave the table "a little hungry." Lori describes her dad as a controlling person who wants others to hear what he has to say but doesn't stick around to listen to their points of view. Although there are many disagreements in their family, they are not outwardly discussed.

Lori began to diet while she was on vacation with her family. She met a female relative a few years older than she who was very thin and fashionable, and who wore make up. Just like her mother, the relative also talked about how important it was to diet and refrain from eating a lot. She had a definite impact on Lori because she epitomized everything her mom had been telling her. It was during this trip that Lori became upset with her parents and refused to eat. Surprisingly, she found that she actually liked the feeling of not eating and, although she was hungry, she enjoyed these new sensations of flying and feeling as if she were empty. She ate less and less on the trip and, as a result, her parents began to pay more attention to her, which also pleased her. For the first time she felt as if she had control over herself and her family. Her control surrounded eating issues and, at one point during her trip, she told her dad that the more he demanded she eat, the less she would eat. However, no matter what her parents did, whether it was ignoring her eating habits or yelling at her to eat more, she continued to limit her food intake, became obsessed with food, and eventually ended up in the hospital due to severe weight loss and malnourishment secondary to her anorexia nervosa (Gottlieb 2000).

HOW ANOREXIA STARTS

Anorexia usually begins in the course of a diet, although those who develop it don't start out thinking that they are going to lose more than their initial target weight. Many with a history of anorexia have said, however, that they didn't feel totally "right" about themselves even before they began to diet. Family members noticed a change before the onset of anorexia also, as some recalled that their children began to separate themselves from friends and family even before the weight loss began. Ari remembers thinking she had to eat healthier to perform better on the tennis team. In addition, many anorexics recall a particular remark, look, or event which made them feel fat, even if they weren't overweight. Experts say that, no matter what the anorexic's actual weight is at the onset of the illness, it is this "last straw" that tips them over and leads to the beginning of their weight loss. Obviously, the memorable event is not truly the cause of the illness but the point at which everything the affected individuals are feeling and thinking that comes to a head. It is the time that they cannot handle any more pressure, conflict, uncertainty, or anxiety within themselves and must find a way to control themselves and their inner anxieties.

In addition to a seemingly benign remark, there are other significant events which are particularly stressful and are known to trigger the onset of anorexia, a recurrence, or at the very least, a preoccupation with weight in some individuals. These events include starting high school or college, moving to a new town or away from home, starting a new job, or even going to camp. One girl's illness started when she travelled alone to Europe for the first time. Another girl's anorexia began when she filled out college applications. Also, traumatic events, such as the death of a parent or sexual abuse can also predate the onset of anorexia. For example, one girl who had been sexually abused when she was younger developed anorexia during puberty when boys began to notice her. Some of these occasions represent the time when adolescents and young adults must prove themselves and demonstrate their independence, when they must show they can be self-reliant, and when they are critiqued by others. They may not feel mentally prepared for such major changes, or they may not want a change to occur (Landau 1983). Many therapists think that individuals who develop anorexia are afraid of becoming adults where they must rely on themselves and make their own decisions. Therefore, during puberty, when their bodies begins to change and they develop adult-like bulges on their hips, legs, and breasts, these individuals lose weight so they can look like a child again. Symbolically, they are delaying the onset of adolescence and the inevitable physical and emotional responsibilities of adulthood.

FOUR STAGES OF ANOREXIA NERVOSA

Steve Levenkron, a psychiatrist who specializes in eating disorders, has broken the development and progression of anorexia into four distinct stages. The first is the achievement stage. Many people enter this phase. They begin to diet and decide they are going to lose a certain amount of weight so that they will look better. Few reach their ultimate goal and fewer remain there. It is different for those who develop anorexia. Their illness almost always starts with a diet. At first their obvious success at losing weight is rewarded by others with praise, awe, and envy. Friends and family make comments about how the individual has lost weight and looks great. Ari said that, even when she told others she had anorexia, they continued to admire her body. One relative even watched her eat and told her that she was going to "copy me exactly because she loved how cute and skinny I was." Some ask how she did it, and others state that they have never had the willpower to go on a diet and stick with it. Once the dieter has surpassed the initial weight loss goal, however, the weight loss continues and the individual begins to think about weight loss all the time. They feel good about themselves, at least in this aspect of their lives. They decide that being hungry is a small price to pay for the sense of achievement. Ari said that she did not notice her suffering but, instead felt great pride about her determination and ability to resist food. She developed very strict and rigid rules regarding her eating, surviving mainly on cut-up apples.

In stage 2, the security-compulsive stage, the individuals have reached their initial weight loss goals. Instead of stopping here, however, they begin to increase their weight loss efforts and develop a new goal, around two pounds a week. Yet, this time there is no end in sight. They become obsessed with measuring every part of their body. The thinner they are, the fatter they feel, increasing their desire to lose more weight. They think of nothing else and begin to ignore or disregard all other aspects of their lives. They no longer have time for friends, family, or extracurricular activities, and they begin to separate themselves from others. They eat fewer and fewer calories and increase the intensity of their exercise. The only thing that makes them feel good is losing weight, and even this feeling of accomplishment is only momentary. They can always lose more weight, can always be thinner. Ari recalls when her eating and exercise level dramatically changed. "I was playing tennis about five times a week and replacing chips with pretzels, but things became extreme quickly. I began to go on the tennis courts every day for hours; I did not care who I played against as long as I was running in place and burning hundreds of calories. Soon my level of play began to decrease because I decided that being skinny was much more important."

In stage 3, the assertive stage, anorexics continues to lose weight, and friends and family begin to tell them that they have lost too much and need to stop dieting. Anorexics think, however, that others are envious of their thinness and success at losing weight. Anorexics, who are typically nice, agreeable, and compliant, often become defiant for the first time in their lives and refuse to stop their weight loss efforts. Although their defiance may only pertain to this aspect of their life, it becomes all-consuming. They no longer feel the need to please others, as they had in the past, and begin to make demands surrounding eating. Some anorexics, for example, may make others leave the kitchen so they can eat alone, or agree to sit at the table for dinner only if nobody comments on what and how much they eat. Their families, who will do anything to ensure that the anorexic eats, comply with the new, rigid orders. Anorexics feel powerful for the first time ever and as if they have some control over their lives. They may try to hide their weight loss by wearing baggy clothes so that others do not try to sabotage their efforts. Ari, who had previously been very loving and caring toward her family, distinctly remembers this stage of her anorexia. "I became hostile toward everyone else, especially my family. I ignored people and gave simple, one-word answers. I avoided all contact with other people and I locked myself in my room all day. I even shut out my pets."

In stage 4, the pseudo-identity stage, anorexics take on a totally different identity and feel a new sense of power and accomplishment; they think they finally have a worthwhile goal in their lives, which is losing weight. Their disease begins to define their identities, and it becomes part of all their relationships and achievements. They often sacrifice other achievements for success in controlling their weight. The longer they have this new identity the more difficult it is to relinquish it and return to a more typical life which is filled with uncertainties. This is a major reason that it is easier to treat those who have had anorexia for a shorter period of time.

What It Feels Like to Be Anorexic

No matter who develops anorexia, whether it is a male, a female, an African American, or a Caucasian, once they develop the illness the thoughts and behaviors that accompany the weight loss become similar. Anorexics don't look at food the way someone without an eating disorder does. Anorexics are always trying to lose weight, always trying to become thinner. There is no end in sight, as there is with someone who diets but then stops dieting once the weight goal is reached. For anorexics, calorie counting becomes irrational to the point that, even eating a single grape can cause much anxiety and distress. Anorexics become obsessed with weight loss and avoid most food groups. Although they feel pangs of hunger, they are willing to ignore or suppress them. Ari recalls these feelings. "If I ate one extra bite of food, I would have to skimp on every single meal for two straight days to feel comfortable in my body again. The terrifying part of the disease is that I was positive that I was gaining fat on my body."

Anorexics begin to refrain from social situations that involve food and may actually ask friends if eating is involved. They don't want to risk any temporary regression in their attempts to lose weight. Characteristically, anorexics tend to be perfectionists and are very driven. They successfully organize every aspect of their lives to help achieve their goal of weight loss. Their identity and self-worth becomes a direct reflection of their ability to become thinner. Some anorexics say that they enjoy feeling hungry and having an empty stomach because it makes them feel thinner. When they feel thinner, they feel good about themselves and in greater control of their lives. Plus, they fear gaining weight more than they fear being hungry. This is exemplified in a statement made by Stella, a 17-year-old with anorexia. "When I was able to lose weight and keep it off, I finally felt as though I was in charge of my own welfare. It was strange, but wonderful—a sort of powerful feeling. I felt as though now I was allowed to please myself" (Landau 1983).

As anorexics lose more weight, they eat less and less. One anorexic ate two crème-filled cookies a day, but eventually decreased her intake to one without the crème (Landau 1983). Another anorexic thought it was absolutely fine to have one cheerio for breakfast. Yet another thought she was gorging if she had more than one peanut butter cracker (Bruch 1973). Everything that touches an anorexic's mouth is thought of in terms of calories, even a postage stamp. Anorexics go to extreme measures to make a small amount of food last a long time, such as by cutting a cookie into sixteen pieces and eating one piece an hour.

ANOREXICS FEEL MORE IN CONTROL OF THEIR LIVES

While family and friends may think that anorexics are out of control and worry that they are dangerously thin, anorexics feels completely "in control," and have a sense of achievement, possibly for the first time in their lives. Laurie, a 17-year-old anorexic said "I just felt fat. Usually in the past I had found it very difficult to control my weight. But now somehow I firmly believed that if I could control my weight, then I would be able to control the rest of my life, and then things would finally go right for me" (Landau 1983). Someone with anorexia may feel physically and morally superior, as if they are doing a better job at something than others, and that others may actually be envious. Anorexics feel important and feel as if they are doing something worthwhile. Hilde Bruch thought that all anorexics expect something "special" for successfully starving themselves and losing weight. The longer they starve themselves successfully, the more special and unique they feel, and the less they interact with others. Their entire world is engulfed by weight loss and how to achieve it. When anorexics are questioned about their weight, they will most likely appear totally unaware of how thin they actually are and will be unwilling to accept that there is anything wrong or different about them. It is likely that they will deny that they have a problem. In fact, they may become upset with someone who doesn't understand their goal or who tries to tell them that they are too thin because they think that the opposite is true—they are too fat.

WEIGHT LOSS LEADS TO ABNORMAL THINKING
AND BEHAVIOR

Anorexics not only feel more in control as they lose weight, but they also feel as if their lives have been simplified and are less overwhelming. In some ways, they are right because starvation actually leads to abnormal thinking and behavior. These changes characteristically occur when someone falls to about 70% to 80% of their ideal body weight, at which point thinking becomes much more rigid. Issues which were once confusing and had many possible paths now appear to be black and white, so it much easier to make a decision. For an anorexic, a situation or issue is right or wrong, good or bad.

In terms of their weight, anorexics are either fat or thin, are eating or aren't eating. They gain further control of their lives by juggling fewer activities than they had previously. Since they spend their days preoccupied with themselves and their weight, other issues become unimportant. As long as they can continue to satisfy their eating and weight requirements, they feel good. School and academic goals, extracurricular activities, and social lives take a back seat or even become nonexistent and they begin to fail in these areas of their lives. The more weight they lose the more rigid and inflexible they become. Interestingly, these rigid behaviors and thoughts begin to disappear when anorexics regain some weight (Slade 1984).

In addition to developing rigid thinking, those who starve themselves also begin to act in strange ways. The new, bizarre behaviors are similar to those exhibited by others who have lost a significant amount of weight. Anorexics become obsessed with all aspects of food, and many begin to cook elaborate meals for others, including family members and friends. They may buy new cookbooks or check them out at the library and pick several new recipes, all of them highly caloric. Often the recipes are very complicated and time consuming. Although they don't eat any of the food themselves, they insist that other family members do. Sometimes parents or siblings complain that, while the anorexic is losing weight, they are gaining. Anorexics often make peculiar meals for themselves, keeping their concoctions very low in calories and fat, such as a mixture of mustard and vinegar.

An interesting experiment was done which demonstrated that, whereas the reasons for starvation may differ, once a person reaches a certain percentage below his IBW, the behaviors become similar to others who are also starving. In this study, soldiers spent six months eating about 1500 calories a day, not enough to maintain their current weight. As they lost more and more weight, they became increasingly obsessed with food. Eventually they began to read cookbooks, buy cooking supplies, and cook for others. They also became antisocial, lost their libido, and developed a very rigid way of thinking. Some become hyperactive. They also lost their self-esteem and began to dislike themselves. Some even began to binge and purge. These behaviors, which occurred as a result of significant weight loss, are similar to the behavioral changes that anorexics have when they lose a significant amount of weight (Slade 1984).

EXERCISE IS AN IMPORTANT COMPONENT OF ANOREXIA

Many people with anorexia also exercise to increase their weight loss. They may keep adding more exercises to their daily routine until they are only sleeping a few hours a night. One teen girl swam up to six hours a day.

Another anorexic walked to and from school, exercised two to three hours after school, and then did jumping jacks for hours when she was supposed to be asleep (Bruch 1973). Some anorexics feel they must constantly move their bodies so they can continue to burn calories, even if it is merely moving a toe back and forth when they are sitting or studying. According to several studies, both sexes use exercise to increase their weight loss, although males are more likely to use it as a major method of weight loss. For example, Dr. Thomas Holbrook, a psychiatrist and recovered anorexic, exercised up to 20 hours a day for years.

BINGING AND PURGING

Although their goal is to remain in control, about 50% of anorexics eventually lose weight by binging and purging. This is in contrast to people with bulimia, where 100% binge and purge while typically maintaining a normal body weight. Marci, an anorexic, consumed six or seven pounds of chocolate; or a cherry cheesecake, a seven-layer cake, and a quart of ice cream; or five or six jars of peanut butter during a single binge (Landau 1983). Another anorexic reported eating seven to eight loaves of bread at one sitting. Not only do anorexics eat exorbitant amounts of food during a binge, but they can also exhibit strange behaviors to support their binges, such as stealing food, rummaging through garbage cans, shoplifting food, or secretly eating leftovers from others' plates (Slade 1984). After the binging episode is over, however, anorexics panic. They are afraid that everything they just ate is going to make them very fat, that they won't be able to lose all the weight they just gained, or that the food will harm them in some other way. Some immediately begin an extreme starvation or liquid diet. Others make themselves vomit, either manually or by using medication. They may use their fingers or an object such as a feather or something else to tickle their throats, which can be very dangerous. Frequent purging can lead to electrolyte abnormalities which can cause seizures and abnormalities within the heart, in addition to direct trauma from the object used or due to the force of the food being regurgitated.

Anorexics may feel ashamed and humiliated after they vomit or, alternatively, they may develop a sense of satisfaction and increased control with the ability to empty their system so efficiently. They are usually very secretive about their vomiting episodes and find a place where they can safely go to make themselves vomit, whether it is inside their own home or elsewhere. They may repeat these episodes frequently, even daily. Some anorexics feel the need to make themselves vomit every time they eat and they can't think about anything else until they do. Binging and purging can become a large part of their daily routine. Once an anorexic has become accustomed to this cycle, it becomes much more difficult to break.

CONFLICTS RESURFACE WITH WEIGHT GAIN

As anorexics begin to regain their weight and think more clearly, issues which led to their conflict before they developed anorexia resurface and cause conflict once again. They may become depressed or angry, or experience mood swings. They may become anxious because their previously rigid, controlled lives suddenly feel overwhelming and fraught with many decisions which must be made. Dr. Bruch refused to treat anorexics that were below a certain weight because it led to alterations in thoughts and behaviors. She thought that therapy would not be beneficial or successful until they were able to think realistically about the issues that led to their starvation.

Our knowledge of anorexia has grown tremendously. We are aware that it can occur in both genders, in multiple ethnic groups, and in a variety of settings. We also know that when anorexics lose a significant amount of weight, they develop a characteristic set of behaviors which are similar to others with this illness. They become rigid, develop rituals and obsessions regarding food, and sacrifice other areas of their life to focus on their weight loss. Some of these behaviors improve with weight gain, although it is an uphill battle.

5

Medical Complications Associated with Anorexia Nervosa

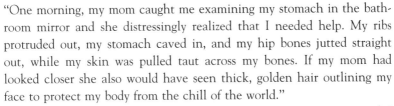

"One morning, my mom caught me examining my stomach in the bathroom mirror and she distressingly realized that I needed help. My ribs protruded out, my stomach caved in, and my hip bones jutted straight out, while my skin was pulled taut across my bones. If my mom had looked closer she also would have seen thick, golden hair outlining my face to protect my body from the chill of the world."

—Ari

When someone loses a lot of weight, whether it is due to anorexia or another reason, the body makes changes to protect itself. Some changes are short-term while others are more chronic (see Figure 5.1). For example, one of the most important things the body does is to stop performing unnecessary jobs so that it can save energy for vital functions. It is this process which can damage organs and, eventually, may inhibit an organ from functioning at all. In anorexics, organs may not only be harmed because of self-starvation, but can also malfunction because of abuse of medicines which are used to try to increase weight loss.

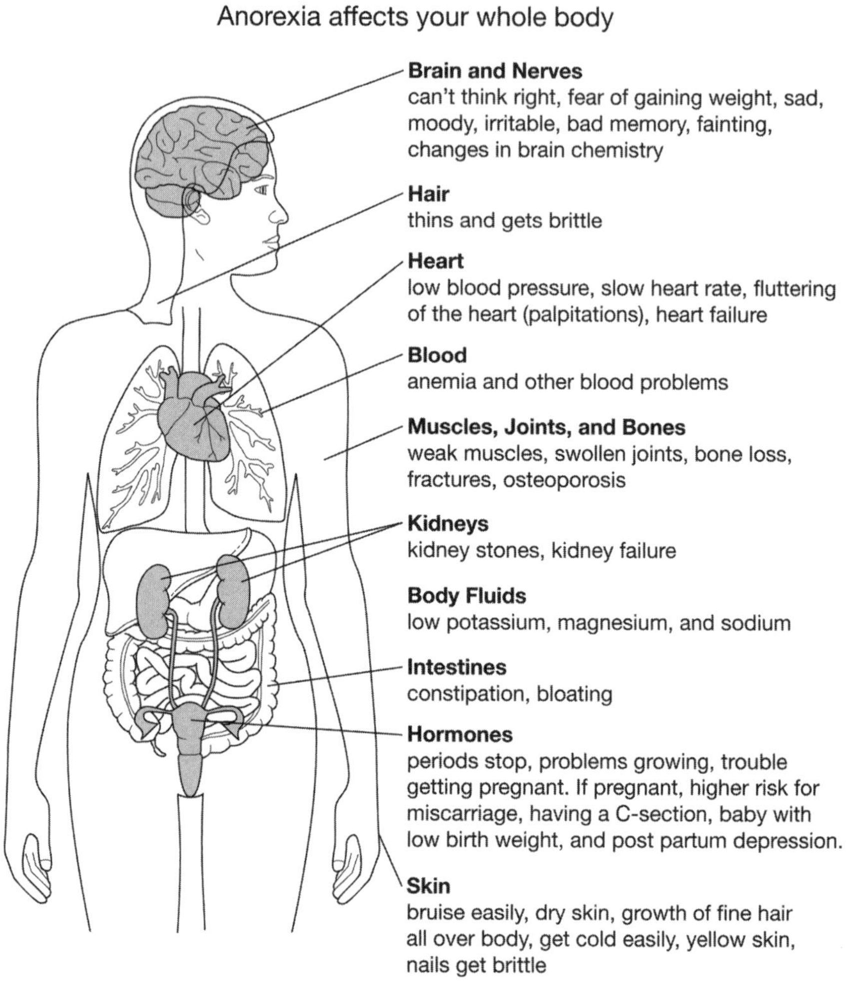

Anorexia affects your whole body

Brain and Nerves
can't think right, fear of gaining weight, sad, moody, irritable, bad memory, fainting, changes in brain chemistry

Hair
thins and gets brittle

Heart
low blood pressure, slow heart rate, fluttering of the heart (palpitations), heart failure

Blood
anemia and other blood problems

Muscles, Joints, and Bones
weak muscles, swollen joints, bone loss, fractures, osteoporosis

Kidneys
kidney stones, kidney failure

Body Fluids
low potassium, magnesium, and sodium

Intestines
constipation, bloating

Hormones
periods stop, problems growing, trouble getting pregnant. If pregnant, higher risk for miscarriage, having a C-section, baby with low birth weight, and post partum depression.

Skin
bruise easily, dry skin, growth of fine hair all over body, get cold easily, yellow skin, nails get brittle

Figure 5.1. How Anorexia Affects Your Body. This illustration shows how anorexia can negatively affect many systems within your body. Illustration by Jeff Dixon.

SIGNIFICANT CHANGES IN MANY HORMONE LEVELS

One organ, or organ system, which begins to function differently because of severe weight loss, is the endocrine system. This system is responsible for releasing hormones and maintaining the body's metabolism. In response to starvation, it begins to alter the levels of many hormones in order to lower the body's metabolism. For example, decreases in levels of hormones which are stored in a special organ in the brain, called the pituitary gland, cause a drop in the core body temperature, heart rate, blood pressure, metabolic rate, and conduction of the heart rhythm. If these changes are severe enough, the anorexic may need to be hospitalized. Second, the levels of sex hormones within the pituitary gland, including luteinizing hormone and follicular stimulating hormone, also drop. Consequently, the male testes produce less testosterone, and the female ovaries make less estrogen. Females with anorexia have a further drop in estrogen levels when they lose weight because they have fewer fat cells, which secrete small amounts of estrogen. All of these changes lead to amenorrhea in females and the loss of libido in both men and women. They also cause a delay in the onset of puberty. In addition, starvation also increases the level of the stress hormone, cortisol, and decreases the effect of growth hormone on growing bones, so that an anorexic will not grow tall as quickly as peers. Typically, all of these changes begin to occur when someone has lost about 15% of their ideal body weight. However, it can take place sooner in an obese individual who has lost a significant amount of weight but has not yet fallen below their IBW.

LOWER LEVELS OF RED AND WHITE BLOOD CELLS

Anorexics also develop other problems as a result of their weight loss. For example, poor nutrition and lack of iron or folate in the diet can lead to anemia, which causes lethargy and weakness. Severe anemia can cause the heart to malfunction. Anorexics can also develop anemia from a generalized "shut down" of the bone marrow, the place where red blood cells are made. In addition to red blood cells, platelets and white blood cells are also produced in the bone marrow. Thus, when it begins to shut down, it not only makes fewer red blood cells, but it also produces fewer platelets, which help clot blood, and fewer white blood cells, which fight off infections. Approximately one-third to two-thirds of patients have some degree of bone marrow malfunction. Although a lower white blood cell count doesn't usually increase the chances that an anorexic may develop an infection or become sick, it can lead to serious problems and even death once an infection develops (Evans et al. 2007). This is partly because someone who has a low white blood cell count and becomes ill may not be able to "mount a response," or show the usual signs and symptoms of an infection, such as a fever or a high white count. Therefore, neither the anorexic nor family and friends may be aware that the anorexic is sick or that the illness is serious. Consequently, treatment may begin too late in the course of the illness. In addition, once an infection occurs it may become more serious in an anorexic because there are fewer white blood cells to fight it off. Several years ago a well-known 21-year-old Brazilian model, Ana Carolina Reston, developed an overwhelming infection secondary to her anorexia and died in the hospital.

MUSCLE AND PROTEIN BREAKDOWN

Starvation can also lead to muscle loss and weakness. After anorexics use all available fat from their fat cells, their bodies look for other sources of energy. One new source is muscle, so the body begins to break it down. As more muscle is used for energy, anorexics lose the ability to exercise as well and their endurance decreases. Muscle loss occurs in all areas of the body, including the heart and intestines. Therefore, it not only affects the ability to exercise, but also the ability of the heart and gastrointestinal tract to function properly (Slade 1984). According to Ari, exercise became much harder with time.

> Even though I ran five miles every day, each week running became harder and harder because my whole body was weakening. I used to feel pressure in my knee caps as if the bones were about to burst through the paper-thin layer of skin. My legs often buckled under me and I would collapse, but I laughed it off and commented on how clumsy I was. I often had pains shooting through my heart that were so painful they would take my breath away.

This widespread muscle loss can lead to cardiomyopathy, or an enlarged, weakened, and ineffective heart. It can also cause difficulty passing stool because the muscles in the intestines are unable to coordinate or effectively push stool toward the rectum. The constipation can be severe, not only because of the weakened muscle, but also for other reasons. First, because an anorexic eats and drinks so little, the body reabsorbs any fluids it can, even from the intestines, resulting in stools that are small, hard pellets. Second, if an anorexic abuses laxatives, such as Metamucil or Colace, the body responds by getting rid of any extra fluid available. This also leads to dehydrated stools in the intestines. Over time the body becomes tolerant and resistant to a specific laxative dose. Thus, larger amounts are needed to achieve similar results, and the anorexic becomes more constipated (National Eating Disorders Association n.d.). In fact, anorexics have been known to take as many as 100 laxatives a day (Slade 1984).

ABUSE OF MEDICATIONS THAT CAN DAMAGE THE BODY

In addition to constipation, laxative abuse can cause other problems as well, some of which are life-threatening. Anorexics often use laxatives after they binge because they think it will rid their bodies of food and fluid that they just consumed and, therefore, calories. Yet laxatives only successfully eliminate water, essential electrolytes (such as sodium and potassium), minerals, and some indigestible fiber. Weight loss from this method is temporary because, when someone drinks again, the body will reabsorb necessary fluid back into the body. If, on the other hand, an anorexic doesn't drink enough fluids, several serious problems can occur, including severe dehydration, electrolyte imbalances, organ failure, and even death. Electrolyte imbalances can significantly interfere with normal functioning of the heart, nerves, and brain. Likewise, if someone suddenly stops using laxatives, their heart and nerves may not function normally because their body is retaining too much water and sodium. Therefore, when stopping the use of a laxative or diuretic, it is important to slowly decrease the medication dose under the guidance of a physician.

Laxative abuse is not the only way an anorexic develops electrolyte abnormalities. Shifts in the fluid and electrolyte balance within the body can also occur when one makes oneself vomit, a process called purging, or when somebody abuses diuretics, medicines that remove excess water from the body. Recurrent purging may lead to low potassium which, in turn, can cause a rapid heart rate, abnormal heart rhythms (arrhythmias), muscle weakness, kidney problems, and the inability of the intestines to function properly. A low sodium level, due to dehydration from any of the means noted above, can lead to mental confusion and seizures. A low phosphate level, caused by diuretic abuse or sudden, rapid refeeding can cause kidney failure, abnormal heart rhythms, and mental confusion. A low magnesium level, sometimes seen with diuretic abuse or severe malnutrition, can also cause cardiac arrhythmias or, alternatively, decrease the body's potassium level. Any of these events can lead to death (Silber 2005).

PROBLEMS WITH THE HEART, STOMACH, AND INTESTINES

As noted above, any combination of muscle loss, electrolyte disturbances, dehydration and weight loss can cause problems within the heart, including, malfunctioning heart valves, arrhythmias, low electrical voltage within the heart, and heart enlargement. Additionally, ipecac, a medication some anorexics use to make themselves vomit, can lead to an irreversible cardiomyopathy, where the heart muscle doesn't work as well as it should. Other complications can arise when anorexics purge (see Chapter 3). Food products and stomach acids that are forcibly regurgitated into the esophagus can cause either a rupture of the stomach or a tear in the esophagus. Purging can also cause an acute enlargement of the stomach, which may lead to death. In addition, chronic purging leads to enlargement of the parotid glands, dental problems due to erosion of the enamel from acid reflux, and chipped, exposed teeth.

NEUROLOGIC PROBLEMS

There are many neurologic problems that can occur as a result of anorexia. For example, anorexics often have sleep problems, including frequent night awakenings and restless, fitful sleep. Despite these restless nights, they are often described as hyperactive and report feeling more energetic than they did before the onset of anorexia. Over time, however, as their weight loss becomes extreme, the increased energy level is replaced by a generalized weakness and fatigue. Another significant neurologic change that occurs is a structural change within the brain. Researchers who have examined brain scans of individuals with and without anorexia have found that anorexics have a dilation, or enlargement of the ventricles, which is the area of the brain where the spinal fluid flows. Researchers have also described atrophy, or shrinking of the white matter, which is the part of the brain used for higher functioning. Experts postulate that this may account for the anorexic's organic brain syndrome, which includes a poorer performance on standardized tests and tests of attention, memory, concentration, and visuospatial ability, when compared to people without anorexia (Treasure, Schmidt, and Van Furth 2003). Many, but not all of these deficits improve after weight and eating patterns return to normal.

Another predictable change which may be neurologic in nature is related to personality. It is interesting that, as anorexics reach a weight which is about 65% of their ideal body weight, their personalities change in similar ways. They become much more obsessed about losing weight and may actually begin to increase the amount of weight they lose each week. In addition, their fear of losing control escalates as does the amount of weight they lose each week. These behavioral changes, particularly the obsession with weight loss, improve as weight increases. Other neurologic changes seen in anorexia include clumsiness with an increased risk of falling, seizures, and a peripheral neuropathy, which is damage to the nerves outside the brain and spinal cord (Slade 1984).

THINNING OF THE BONES

Common side effects which occur after starvation for six months or longer are osteopenia, or a decrease in bone mass, and osteoporosis, which is actual bone loss. These problems occur in almost one-half of anorexics. While adolescence is usually the time when bone is forming and bone mass is increasing the most, the opposite occurs with anorexics. This is because calcium and phosphate, which are the building blocks of bones, are being removed from the bone to be used for essential functions in other areas of the body. Additionally, low estrogen in females and low testosterone in males, worsen the osteoporosis. Furthermore, excessive exercise leading to amenorrhea, and elevated cortisol levels also promote bone loss. Once osteoporosis or osteopenia has occurred, the risk of developing fractures, having delayed healing of a fracture, or of developing severe, chronic bone pain significantly increases. Ari fractured her foot during the height of her anorexia and remembers that it took awhile to heal. She also recalls severe injuries from minor incidents, such as the need to use crutches after she sprained her ankle. Anorexics need to be within about 10% of their IBW to inhibit further bone loss, although they never completely recover the loss which took place during their illness and, consequently, have a much higher risk of developing fractures and chronic pain even years after recovery. While researchers are trying to find ways to improve bone density, including hormone replacement therapy, they have not been very successful yet.

COMPLICATIONS OF ANOREXIA NERVOSA IN ADULTHOOD

Even years after being diagnosed with anorexia, adults continue to suffer the psychological effects of their illness. According to a study done by psychiatrist David Herzog, about one-third of people who had been diagnosed with anorexia are doing well or have no problems as adults, about one-third still have some issues surrounding eating and body image issues with intermittent eating disorder symptoms, and one-third still have anorexia or have developed bulimia (Silber 2009). Those with a history of anorexia are also more likely to have problems with sexual relationships and fertility, the ability to become pregnant as adults. In fact, there is as much as a two-thirds decrease in fertility. If these adults do become pregnant, they have a greater risk of spontaneous abortion, twice the risk of delivering a baby early, and a greater likelihood that they will need a cesarean section, even if they aren't currently diagnosed with a disorder. These problems may arise from continued issues surrounding food, resulting in persistent malnutrition, low weight in the pregnant mother and child, and abnormal hormone levels. As a result of the mothers' problems, their newborns are also more likely to have a medical complication. For example, infants who are born prematurely are six times more likely to die within the first few weeks of birth than those born at term (Treasure, Schmidt, and Van Furth 2003). Also, babies who are born with a low birth weight are at a greater risk of having difficulty feeding and of developing a serious infection.

While pregnancy is difficult for someone with current or past anorexia, being a new mom can also be difficult and stressful. As soon as their babies are born, new mothers have to learn how to take care of and feed them. Moms not only worry about how much to feed their newborns, but they also worry about their own weight and body shape. Once they have given birth, they think that they no longer have a valid reason for carrying around the extra weight they gained during pregnancy. This can lead to a recurrence of abnormal eating behaviors and/or postpartum depression. Some women will obsess about their weight gain and spend so much time and effort thinking about and trying to lose it that they don't bond with or give enough time to their newborns. Then when they don't spend time with their newborns, they feel guilty (Gura 2007).

Each transition in a child's life can lead to feelings of guilt and the resurgence of anorexia in the mother. Not only may these women have daily difficulties regarding their eating and weight issues, but they may also have them with regard to their children. Whether it is deciding how much food to give an infant or toddler, packing snacks for a school-age child, or making cupcakes for a birthday party, a child's life is surrounded by food. Studies have shown that mothers with anorexia are more likely than mothers without anorexia to misperceive their children as being overweight when they aren't. In addition, mothers with eating disorders are more likely to think their children are pudgy or greedy eaters when they are not. In some cases, these children are actually malnourished. Furthermore, children whose mothers are anorexic are more likely to be obsessed with food and weight than children whose mothers don't have anorexia. In a study of 5,331 adolescent girls and 3,881 adolescent boys and their mothers, those who said weight was more important to their mother, and were correct, were more frequently obsessed about thinness and had dieted. Some teens who know their mother has eating issues will use food as a form of rebellion. Trisha Gura, author of *Lying in Weight*, retells the story of Ethan, whose mom has alcoholism, anorexia, and bulimia. Ethan did not think his mom was adequately concerned about his abuse of drugs, alcohol, and cigarettes. When he realized, however, that her major concern was his weight, he began to use it as a form of rebellion. While she repeatedly told him she wanted him to be thin and in shape, he became obese and finally got a response for which he was searching (Gura 2007).

Adults with a history of anorexia have other problems as well. Psychologically, they continue to have rigid personalities, making it more difficult for them to succeed in their endeavors and, when they are successful, they often don't feel satisfied. People who had anorexia for several years and those who currently have it have spent so much time focusing on weight loss that they haven't concentrated on their education or work opportunities and, consequently, are limited in what they can do. Many have dreams that were never fulfilled and fewer life choices and activities. Their social networks and friends are limited and they often have sexual problems in their intimate relationships. Their family interactions have changed, and they often feel guilt and shame.

RECOVERY AND PROGNOSIS

Just as there is debate surrounding the exact diagnosis of anorexia nervosa, there is also disagreement about what should constitute "recovery" in someone with anorexia. Some think recovery should be defined as the elimination of every symptom of anorexia. Others, however, think anorexics have recovered when they don't meet all the criteria required for diagnosis for a certain time period. The problem with the latter definition is that, even though some people don't meet all the criteria for anorexia, they may still have significantly abnormal thoughts or behaviors regarding their weight, diet, and/or body image. There is also debate about the length of time someone should be symptom-free before they are considered recovered. In some studies, a remission is defined as eight weeks without symptoms, while in others it is defined as a year. People tend to regain their weight well before they recover psychologically, sometimes by as much as a year. Ari specifically mentioned this in one her essays when she stated, "My body recovered much faster than my mind." As noted earlier, this mind-body discrepancy was noted by Dr. Hilde Bruch, who stated that anorexics would not be able to participate in therapy or respond appropriately if their weight was too low (Bruch 1978). One possible way to reduce the discrepancies is by using two terms, remission and recovery, when discussing improvement after having anorexia.

No matter what definition is used to define recovery, we know that it is a difficult road for those with anorexia and that many who have this illness never completely recover. Ari points out the complexity and constant turmoil she had during her own recovery.

Each day of recovery is a little easier, but I still battle the world to function for just one day. Mornings are extremely difficult because I am always emotional . . . I feel so bad because I am so against gaining weight and seeing my body change, but at the same time a part of me wants the fat. It is hard having a constant conflict in your head all day and night, especially because I am such a passive person.

The younger the anorexic and the more quickly the illness is diagnosed after its onset, the better the chances of partial or complete improvement.

Young adolescents who have anorexia and recover relatively quickly have a better chance of developing a normal personality and a positive self-esteem than those who have it as older teens and adults (Berkman, Lohr, and Bulik 2007). The latter group is more likely to be cautious and anxious and have a low sense of autonomy and effectiveness. They are also more likely to be diagnosed with personality disorders, such as an avoidant, dependent, or obsessive-compulsive disorder, even years after they have been diagnosed with and received treatment for anorexia.

Besides age and amount of time one has the illness, other issues also factor into the overall prognosis. One study showed that hospitalized anorexics who were motivated to change and were willing to take the steps necessary to reach their goals were more likely to maintain their healthier weights after they left the hospital (Castro-Fornieles et al. 2006). Additionally, patients who are able to develop a good, therapeutic relationship with their therapist also do better than those who don't. Anorexics who exercise excessively tend to have longer inpatient stays and relapse quicker than those who don't (Shroff et al. 2006).

Statistics regarding prognosis and outcome depend on how a study is conducted. First, as mentioned previously, they depend on how researchers define recovery in that particular study. Second, the results depend on how many years after the diagnosis a study is conducted. For example, results four years after a diagnosis of anorexia is made will most likely be different than results obtained 10 years after diagnosis. In fact, depending on the criteria used, studies have shown that the percentage of anorexics who have recovered four years after diagnosis ranges anywhere from 0 to 92%.

According to one study, the median time it took from developing physical symptoms to recovery was 57 months, while recovery from the psychological symptoms took 79 months (Couturier and Lock 2006a). Research recently conducted on patients who were admitted into a hospital for treatment of anorexia showed that, 12 years after their hospitalization, about 33% still had the diagnosis of anorexia nervosa, either due to the chronic nature of the illness or to a recurrence. Ten percent were diagnosed with another disorder, bulimia. The risk of death was greater than 10% (Fichter, Quadflieg, and Hedlund 2006). A literature review, based on 62 outcome studies, documented that five years after diagnosis, 50% of anorexics had recovered, 6% still had the diagnosis of anorexia, 22% had been diagnosed with bulimia nervosa, and 14% had EDNOS. Ten years after diagnosis, 27% had an eating disorder (Berkman, Lohr, and Bulik 2007). Another review article looked at different variables to see how patients did long-term. They reported that 24% of patients had recovered in all areas of functioning at follow up, including actual weight, eating patterns, body image, social adjustment, and resumption of menses. Another 26% had a good outcome with full recovery of weight and menstruation but with some persistent body image disturbances or disordered eating. About 31% had partially recovered some of their weight but hadn't resumed normal menses and still had some psychological issues. Twelve percent had a poor outcome, and 7% had died (Gordon 2000).

The long-term prognosis for someone diagnosed with anorexia is discouraging, to say the least. Years later, many are still having problems and almost one-third continue to meet criteria for an eating disorder, whether it is anorexia nervosa or has moved into the category of bulimia nervosa. Plus, the risk of dying is the highest of any mental illness. Studies have indicated that the mortality rate can reach 20% within 20 years after being diagnosed with anorexia (Silber 2005). The major causes of death are starvation, suicide, and sudden cardiac death, usually because of electrolyte abnormalities. The suicide rate in women with anorexia is 57 times higher than that of normal women of the same age in the general population (Evans et al. 2007). Other causes of death include tears of the esophagus and ruptures of the stomach due to purging and binging. Infections and chronic organ failure can also result in death, and are a direct result of chronic starvation and medication abuse.

6

Theory of Anorexia and Early Treatments

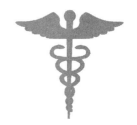

"Mom, there's someone controlling my mind and forcing me to torture myself in worse ways than you can ever imagine."

—Ari

What causes anorexia? We don't know entirely, although the most popular model today combines aspects of many theories, including those based on the biological, psychological, sociological, and cultural perspectives. However, physicians and others have been developing hypotheses and proposing treatments for almost three centuries. As you may recall, in the 1600s Richard Morton, a British physician, provided descriptions of patients with what may be modern-day anorexia nervosa. In his paper *Phthisiologica: or, A Treatise on Consumption*, he discussed a specific group of patients who had wasting but no other obvious medical problems, and he attributed their weight loss to sadness and anxiety, or "atrophia nervosa." In his treatise, Morton writes, "The Causes which dispose the Patient to this Disease, I have for the most part observed to be violent Passions of the Mind, the intemperate drinking of Spirituous Liquors, and an unwholesome Air, by which it is no wonder if the Tone of the Nerves, and thin Temper of the Spirits are destroy'd" (Malson 1998). Morton recommended treatment as soon as possible because he thought that chronic cases were more difficult to cure. His plan may have been the first treatment regimen recommended for someone who starved themselves. It included cheerful discussions, exercise, and spending good times with friends. If this failed, he then recommended fresh country air.

THEORIES AND TREATMENTS DURING THE NINETEENTH CENTURY

Determining the cause of an illness during the nineteenth century was much different than it is today. These days, to test a theory, researchers often design a study with a control and experimental group, identify and isolate a single variable, and evaluate results based on complicated statistical analyses. In addition, other professionals in the field must review the study before it can be published in a reputable journal. In the 1800s, however, theories were not based on such intricate methods but were sometimes decided merely after a period of observation. During this earlier time period, the approach to medicine was holistic, and the overall consensus was that the mind and body greatly affected one another. Physicians and philosophers used the holistic approach particularly when they dealt with women. They thought that ailments which affected a woman's entire body, mind, and spirit originated in a specific organ, the stomach, or gastric center. Later, they added the nervous system as a potential place where emotional and medical illnesses originated. Eventually, physicians merged the gastric center and nervous system together and referred to them collectively as "nervous disorders."

During the 1800s it was fashionable for women to complain of problems in the gastric center and nervous system, which they often did. It was also acceptable for them to appear sickly and to become invalids. They frequently complained that they had colic, abdominal pain, and dyspepsia, or indigestion. They also complained of being nervous or having a nervous disorder. When they had several symptoms related to abdominal pain, they had what was referred to as "hypochondria." Over time, these specific problems became associated with being female. As a result, situations and events specific to women, such as the development of breasts, menstruation, pregnancy, childbirth, and menopause, were all considered pathological and to be potential, likely causes of illnesses, such as nervousness and apepsia, a stomach condition. Words used to describe women and their multiple sickly states included hysteria, neurasthenia, and chlorosis. Dr. M.E. Dirix, a physician in the late nineteenth century, wrote that "women are treated for diseases of the stomach, liver, kidney, heart, lung, etc., yet in most instances, these diseases will be found, on due investigation, to be no disease at all, but merely the symptoms of one disease, namely, a disease of the womb" (Malson 1998).

During that era many prominent physicians tried to find a cause and treatment for the wasting diseases they observed. Although each physician had his own spin on the etiology, the theories were similar to one another because they all involved common assumptions of their period. For example, the two men who were responsible for defining anorexia as a unique disease, Sir William Gull and Charles Laségue, kept within the framework of their time when they contemplated both the cause of and treatment for the illness. Gull wrote that the weight loss in anorexics was secondary to a lack of appetite due to a "perversion of the ego." He was able to surmise that anorexia was not a stomach condition because the food that was eaten had been well digested. In addition, he did not think that it was a symptom of hysteria. However, he chose a common theory of that period when he stated that anorexia occurred because the effected were neurotic. This is why, when contemplating what to label the individuals he described, he recommended dropping the word "apepsia," which had to do with the stomach, and replacing it with "anorexia." In terms of treatment, Gull stated that the afflicted needed good food and nursing because medicine would not work. Appropriate foods included cream, milk, soup, eggs, fish, and chicken to be given in two hour intervals. He also specified that the patients wear heavy clothing and that they receive "warm bed rest" and external heat on the spine. According to Gull, the patient had to be removed from the home environment, particularly family and friends. His treatment recommendations were similar to treatments recommended for a variety of illnesses during that period, which included warm baths, massages, cooking favorite and desirable foods, electric shock, and forced bed rest. Laségue did not comment much on the treatment plan but did write that once the anorexics saw the obvious fear on their families' faces, they would begin to eat again. Laségue, like Gull, used popular theories of that era to define the cause of anorexia. He hypothesized that it was a form of hysteria linked to hypochondriasis and disturbances within the gastric center, which is why he recommended calling the condition "inanition hysterique." The English translation is a hysterical person who is fainting from exhaustion.

Other physicians who cared for these individuals during the 1800s proposed their own theories and treatment recommendations, yet they also developed hypotheses which were consistent with views of that era. For example, the physician Robert Whytt preached that aversion to food was due to problems with the gastric nerves. Louis-Victor Marcé thought that the self-starvation he observed in young teen girls was a type of "hypochondrical delirium," a form of insanity which occurred alongside dyspepsia in girls as they were going through puberty (Silverman 1987b). Dr. Berdt Hovell thought anorexics were physically, emotionally, or morally weakened and recommended encouragement and kindness (Malson 1998). In addition, Pierre Briquet hypothesized that this condition was due to hysteria because of an abnormality within the brain. In terms of treatment recommendations, he suggested that they be surrounded by a pleasant atmosphere, as unpleasant experiences and emotions could worsen the condition.

Marcé developed a detailed treatment plan based on failures of these girls to gain weight at home. He recommended removing them from their homes and placing them under the care of strangers, who would gradually increase their food intake. If there was no place to send the individual, Marcé recommended an asylum, which was not an uncommon place for anorexics to go in the late 1800s. He suggested intimidation and force for those who refused to eat, hoping that these methods could break down even the most stubborn of anorexics. If a patient needed to be force fed, he recommended macerating the food and then spooning, dripping, pushing, or pumping it into the mouth of a patient or, if necessary, placing a tube in the esophagus. Marcé stressed that this condition could be life-threatening and, therefore, needed strong measures. These treatments were advised in the 1880s in the *American Journal of Insanity*. Some families responded well to this plan because they had become so anxious and scared that the parents welcomed the assurance that their child would gain weight. Others, however, feared what effect the intimidation and force would have on their child (Bemporad 1996).

Stuart Chipley, the first American physician to discuss anorexia, agreed with his European colleagues. He thought that food refusal in his patients was merely a "phase of insanity," during which time there was an intense dread of food. In terms of treatment, Chipley recommended placing these girls in an insane asylum to teach them proper moral behavior and to force feed them for the purpose of saving their lives. Reportedly, Chipley not only wanted to admit these girls for their benefit, but also for his own. Since most of them came from middle-class families who were able to pay for hospital stays, Chipley benefitted financially. As he stated, "These cases are remarkable because they are almost peculiar to well-education and sensible people, belonging to the higher walks of society" (Brumberg 2000).

While most physicians continued to use a holistic approach when they thought about the cause of anorexia, some began to think about the brain in new ways. Toward the end of the 1800s, some professionals thought the brain had a specific role in behavior and mental illness, and that other organs, such as the stomach and womb, did not necessarily play a part in these illnesses. One such professional was Dr. Fleury Imbert, a French physician who practiced in the mid-1800s. He hypothesized that the loss of appetite, or "anorexia," was due to the lack of excitement in a specific region within the brain. He also attributed the personality changes he saw in these patients, such as sadness, anger, and fear, to a problem within the "encephalon's grey matter." Although Imbert, like other physicians in the 1800s, assumed that the wasting seen in "anorexia" was due to a loss of appetite rather than the refusal to eat, he was still one of the first to develop this new way of thinking about the brain and mental illnesses.

PSYCHIATRY TO ENDOCRINOLOGY TO PSYCHIATRY: THEORIES IN THE EARLY TWENTIETH CENTURY

By the end of the century, many new and unique hypotheses regarding anorexia were being developed. William Playfair (1835–1903), an English physician, theorized that anorexia could be due to industrialization and improved technology. Psychiatrists, who were seeing more cases of anorexia, began to pay particular attention to the emotional or subconscious component of the illness. In the 1880s, Jean-Martin began to identify different types of anorexia and did not believe that it was a form of hysteria. He thought the patients needed to be isolated because the environment was partly responsible for their problems. One of his pupils, Pierre Janet (1859–1947), a well-known psychiatrist who contributed to the field of psychoanalysis and psychotherapy, hypothesized that anorexia was a psychological problem where the lack of eating was a symptom of a deeper issue. He observed that people with anorexia had many characteristics in common with those who had obsessive-compulsive disorder, including the need to be perfectionists and to obsess about food. Janet did not think that anorexics were revolted by food but rather that they were obsessed with the need to control their own hunger and food intake. In fact, Janet thought that his patients' obsessions were so severe that asking one of them to eat was no different than asking them to urinate in public (Brumberg 2000).

One of Janet's peers was the well-known Sigmund Freud (1856–1939), the founder of psychoanalysis. Although Freud did not spend a considerable amount of time contemplating anorexia, he briefly wrote about it. Freud thought that anorexia was linked to sexuality, and that appetite was directly related to libido and sex drive. He postulated that sexuality was underdeveloped in those with anorexia and that food, or sex, revolted them. More specifically, Freud thought that anorexics didn't eat because they were disgusted by food and its symbolism, rather than because of a desire to control their hunger. In addition, they had a fear of adulthood and sexuality. By not eating, they remained small; their bodies didn't develop or showed regression of secondary sex characteristics, such as breasts and larger testes; and they lost their libido.

The psychoanalytic theories by Freud and others dominated the field of anorexia until 1914, when a pathologist named Morris Simmonds (1855–1925) performed an autopsy on a woman who had exhibited many symptoms similar to those seen in anorexics. He noticed that she had atrophy, or shrinkage, of the anterior pituitary gland (Vandereycken and van Deth 1994). The pituitary gland is an important organ in the brain which secretes hormones that help regulate stress, puberty, menses, thyroid function, metabolism, water regulation, and growth. A deficiency of one or more of these hormones can lead to many problems throughout the body, including severe weight loss. His discovery led to a shift in thinking about the cause of anorexia, and for the next two decades anorexia was considered to be a disease due to abnormal hormone levels. Researchers varied as to which hormone they thought caused the weight loss, with the most common being growth hormone and thyroid hormone. As a result, these hormones were given to anorexics to try to induce weight gain. Researchers at the renowned Mayo Clinic gave thyroid extract to girls who, on blood tests, had a low basal metabolic rate. Unknowingly, they were increasing the thyroid level mostly in people who already had enough, resulting in excess thyroid and, consequently, further weight loss. Occasionally, however, it did cause weight gain, so it became the treatment of choice for several years while other therapies fell out of favor. Other hormones, such as insulin, antuitrin, and estrogen were also given to try to reverse the weight loss, although they were not very effective.

Simmonds' pituitary theory, along with others involving endocrine abnormalities, remained in the forefront of anorexia research until the late 1930s. At this time, physicians learned how to differentiate people with Simmonds' disease from those with other types of wasting, based on their appearance and the results of blood tests. In 1937, and again in 1939, Sheehan was the first to show that being extremely thin was not a consistent or early feature in those with pituitary gland abnormalities. Furthermore, research demonstrated that about half the cases diagnosed as Simmonds' disease were, in actuality, anorexia nervosa. For a brief period, the psychoanalytic models gained prominence again, and decreased food intake was described as a symptom of an unconscious conflict. One of the first well-received theories that surfaced in the early 1940s was the "oral impregnation theory." Several psychiatrists hypothesized that anorexia develops as a result of an oral fixation (the desire to put something in one's mouth, as is done by infants) in individuals who are unable to adapt well to situations. This makes sexual changes that occur during puberty difficult because, in addition to other occasions that cause extreme stress, puberty can

make such an individual want to return to a time where they had oral fulfillment, such as infancy. Thus, when the body begins to develop adult features,
the individual tries to regress toward infancy. Psychoanalysts further hypothesized that anorexics associated eating with becoming pregnant through "oral
impregnation," and that obesity symbolized pregnancy. Such fears led some
individuals to obsess about eating and to repress their sexual wishes and desires.

FAMILY AND ENVIRONMENT: THEORIES IN THE SECOND
HALF OF THE TWENTIETH CENTURY

By the second half of the twentieth century, psychoanalytic theories dimin-
ished in importance and others, which focused on problems within the family,
came into play. Today, certain aspects of these theories continue to be seen as
contributing factors to the development of anorexia. The most prominent theories are those of Mara Selvini Palazzoli, an Italian psychiatrist, and Hilde
Bruch, a psychoanalyst who emigrated from Germany to the United States.
More recently, Gerald Russell has also made important contributions to the
field. Selvini Palazzoli, who wrote extensively in the 1960s, said that a girl
develops anorexia when she is unable to separate her own body from the
image of the "maternal object." Selvini Palazzoli thought that the anorexic's
mother somehow interferes with the girl's ability to become an individual,
which becomes accentuated during puberty. The child, who feels helpless
because she has no identity, tries to gain some sense of control and to protect
herself and, thus, begins to starve herself (Bemporad 1996).

In the 1970s and 1980s, Bruch also characterized those who developed anorexia as feeling helpless and lacking a sense of independence. Bruch hypothesized that family dynamics are involved in the development of anorexia and
that ineffective parenting, where a mother always imposes her own needs on
her children instead of concentrating on her children's needs, leads to the
child's inability to develop a sense of self. Consequently, by the time adolescence arrives, these individuals have lived their entire lives trying to please
others and don't know what they want or need for themselves. They feel
unprepared and cannot cope with the stress of feeling unable to successfully
separate from their families and become a competent adult. They try to gain
some control of themselves and do so by controlling their bodies. Successful
control over their weight provides them with a new feeling of power and comfort, with the additional benefit of giving them control over their family for
the first time rather than the other way around. Furthermore, obsessing about
food allows them to ignore other, more overwhelming aspects of adolescence
and family issues.

Bruch also proposed that anorexics exhibit specific ways of thinking that can lead to the development of anorexia. First, they have an almost delusional, distorted body image, where they think that they are fat even though they aren't. Second, they are confused about and often misinterpret their body's sensations and needs, such as hunger. Third, they feel ineffective and helpless when it comes to their own thoughts and actions because their lives are based on demands and expectations of others. They are often very compliant and, consequently, are praised by adults. Their accommodating lifestyle becomes a problem during adolescence, when teens are expected to develop autonomy and become independent thinkers and doers in preparation for adulthood. Because some individuals do not feel prepared or ready to cope, they become preoccupied with their bodies. Bruch noticed that most individuals who developed anorexia had similar personalities and backgrounds, and that they came from families that stressed achievement and desired perfection. They often placed a high value on superficial appearance and weight control and had a desire to please others. Affected individuals were smart, sensitive, attractive, and usually white females; they were also perfectionists.

Both Bruch and Russell believe that not only has the incidence of anorexia increased, but also that the main cause of the disorder has changed. For that reason, Bruch divided anorexia nervosa into two categories, primary and secondary. Primary anorexia was more common many years ago, when anorexics stopped eating because of a fear they had against sexuality or responsibilities that came with being an adult. She described secondary anorexia as a more recent phenomenon, where a fear of becoming fat has become a greater factor in the development of anorexia. Both believed that the act of reading about anorexia and hearing about it from others may be a new risk factor that didn't exist several decades ago. Bruch thought that girls she treated in therapy who were already familiar with the disease approached it differently. They did not seem to feel the same sense of accomplishment about what they have achieved in terms of weight loss, and they did not place as much emphasis on or feel as unique or superior because of their weight loss as anorexics did years ago. In addition, they did not isolate themselves as much as earlier anorexics, but instead looked for others who were also trying to maintain a waif-like existence.

This second type of anorexic is seen today surfing the Internet to find others with similar goals, responding to self-help groups, asking for help in weight loss efforts, and advising others on how to live life as an anorexic. Support is easily found through one of the many pro-ana Web sites, which promote anorexia as a positive condition and as a choice or lifestyle, rather than an illness. As of September 2007, there were over 500 pro-ana Web sites. Most contain an "Ana creed," such as "I will be thin at all costs, nothing else matters." They also have their "thin commandments," which are a set of rules one can follow to become anorexic. In addition, they commonly offer chat rooms, where participants can talk about their daily diets and get information on how to lose weight quickly. They not only provide support for each other in their attempts to lose weight, but sometimes compete against each other to try to eat the fewest calories or have the greatest weight loss. They may also seek advice on how to purge effectively. Other common components are religious metaphors such as "thinspirations," photos and quotes designed to motivate others in their attempts to lose weight. A review article which examined these Web sites found that the most common themes included control, success, and perfection (Norris et al. 2006). When a group of female anorexics were interviewed about the pro-ana sites, most said they participated in them. They said that involvement in the site helped pass time, made them feel less lonely, gave them advice on tips and tricks, and provided encouragement and support for the lifestyle they have chosen. Researchers evaluated what would happen to nonanorexic college female students after they viewed a pro-ana Web site, as compared to a group that viewed a different Web site about women's fashion. They found that those who viewed the pro-ana site reported a lower self-esteem and more negative view of their own appearance than the other group. They also thought that they were heavier and said that they were more likely to exercise and think about their weight in the near future than the control group (Bardone-Cone and Cass 2007).

SOCIOCULTURAL THEORY

Proponents of the sociocultural theory, another popular theory which has gained attention over the past few decades, believe that our society's current social and cultural views have had a major impact on the incidence of anorexia. This is particularly interesting in light of all the changes that have occurred over the past century. In general, these theorists propose that anorexia nervosa is caused by pressure in Western society to conform to a thin ideal of beauty, or to try to look as we think others in our society want us to look. Historian Caroline Walker Bynum (1941–) considers society and culture to be major factors in the development of anorexia and believes that these factors have influenced women for centuries. She has studied women from prior eras and has hypothesized that those who starved themselves during the Medieval and Renaissance Period for "religious reasons" actually may have done so to escape from cultural conformity. According to Bynum, by starving themselves, these women were able to control themselves and their environment. More specifically, they successfully escaped the cultural norm of a prearranged marriage, the monotonous and unfulfilling life as a wife, and the risk of dying during childbirth. Additionally, they were able to express their displeasure with society in a more acceptable, passive manner.

Further support for this theory comes from the fact that the incidence of anorexia has increased in Western society as the cultural expectations have transformed from one of inner to outer beauty, and as we have greater exposure to magazines, newspapers, television, and movies. Over the past several decades, the entertainment industry has increasingly employed thin role models. In fact, today many models, actresses, and other celebrities are thinner than ever before, often far below their ideal weight. Even children's toys, such as Barbie, provide a depiction of a female that is far too thin. The transformation of our society to one that is obsessed with weight is evident. A large survey done in San Francisco found that 80% of fourth-grade girls were dieting at the time of the survey. Another recent study found that 29% of boys and 41% of girls, ages 8 to 10 years, were trying to control their weight through exercise and diet at the time of the survey (Brumberg 2000). In addition, research has shown that TV and magazines influence women. For example, one study found that more women who looked at slim figures in magazines and on TV thought they were fat and wanted to go on a diet than those who didn't view the figures (Harrison and Cantor 1997). In fact, research indicates that children as young as age 5 years have been concerned about their weight and are afraid of becoming fat.

Yet, although this unrealistic idea of a perfect woman exists in our culture and other Westernized societies, it does not exist worldwide. Those cultures which have not been westernized and have not adopted the notion that thin is beautiful have much lower rates of anorexia than we do. Further, research shows that if someone from a nonwestern society moves to a culture obsessed with being thin, that individual would face an increased risk of developing anorexia.

Levenkron also believes that the fashion industry plays an influential role, especially with women. He postulates that some women hate their bodies because of society's pressure to be thin. This, in combination with the pressure on children and teens to become independent at a much younger age than in the past, is what leads to the development of anorexia. As Brumberg (2000) stated in her book, parental involvement has decreased significantly over the years, from acting as a troop leader in girls' organizations to teaching a child how to use a sanitary napkin. Levenkron thinks that fewer men develop anorexia because they are not sent the same message about weight and body image as women. However, the men who do become ill are more likely to be those who have identified with the message that society has sent to women.

If society and culture alone were responsible for anorexia, then we would expect all individuals who are exposed to the thin ideal to develop this illness. However, this isn't the case. Levenkron thinks these are some of the factors that contribute to its development, but certainly not all. He postulates that children who develop a sense of trust and self-identity are not as vulnerable to the outside culture or external influences. However, children who have not formed their own identity may be looking for it elsewhere, such as in the external environment. He thinks there are several groups at greater risk of developing anorexia. The first are those who undergo traumatic experiences in childhood, such as a divorce, family death, or a chronic illness within the family because any of these can lead to the lack of trust early in life. Because of the inability to trust what their parents say or do, the children don't develop a positive self-esteem or sense of fulfillment, even when they succeed. When adolescence approaches and these children still haven't completed a successful childhood, they begin to look elsewhere for a role model or someone to help them find their own sense of identity. Their search leads them to role models in our society, such as those in the media. They begin to emulate these woman and diet to look more like them. Since they haven't developed a trusting relationship with their parents, they don't believe them when their parents say "enough" to the weight loss and continue to starve themselves.

According to Levenkron, a second group is at increased risk of developing anorexia, because of their inability to form a true, positive identity. This group consists of children who do not hear positive things about themselves and, therefore, assume the negative. If they don't hear they are smart, they will assume they are dumb. If they are not told they are attractive, they will think they are ugly. These children come up with a false sense of who they think they are but don't truly believe this is their identity, so they also search outside their family for their true identity. A third, final group at increased risk of having anorexia consists of children who have mental illnesses, such as depression or anxiety, because they develop a negative view of themselves.

DEVELOPMENTAL THEORY

Arthur Crisp (1930–2006), another renowned psychiatrist in the field of eating disorders, hypothesized that the development of anorexia is due to a combination of biological and psychological experiences which make some individuals feel conflicted about going through puberty and developing an adult body. To them, the adult body signifies the need to deal with adult responsibilities. To prevent this from happening, they diet and starve themselves so they can regress to prepubertal size, developmental level, and life experiences. Crisp explained that there is an intense fear, or phobia, of gaining weight and under-going puberty, more so in females than in males because girls' bodies change more appreciably than boys'. Not only do girls have fat added to their bodies, but they also develop a characteristic adult female shape and begin to menstru-ate. These changes indicate that a female is able to become pregnant, a truly adult responsibility, which can lead to conflict and the desire to be "less fat." Because of their severe phobia of developing an adult body, these individuals will do whatever is possible to avoid food and weight gain. Crisp observed the panic they feel when placed in situations where they must eat, and noted that they feel constant pressure from society and from biological cues to eat. Females who begin and then continue to lose weight during puberty feel a sense of relief, and their intense phobia and sense of panic lessens. To avoid food, the anorectic may adopt strange rituals, abnormal food habits, and avoid social situations where food is available. Because the weight loss brings about a feeling of relief and a sense of protection, the anorectic has no desire to change the current situation.

Crisp thought that certain personality characteristics increase the risk of developing anorexia, including rigidity and avoidance, particularly during peri-ods of stress. He made several treatment recommendations but, most signifi-cantly, stated that the therapist must persuade the patient to admit that she doesn't want to be where she is, biologically and emotionally, and that she wants to change. When her transition begins, she must start at the age level where she currently is psychologically and biologically. For example, she doesn't need to have a target weight set for the age of an adult, but rather the weight she would have during adolescence (Crisp 2006).

ADDICTION THEORY

Some researchers think that anorexia nervosa fits into the model of an addiction, similar to alcohol or drugs. They hypothesize that people with ano-rexia have certain personalities which make them more likely to become ad-dicted to weight loss and exercise. The actual "weight loss" addiction is broken into three stages. The first is the recruitment stage, where the typical diet becomes an obsession. This can occur because of personality traits, body chemistry, or emotional reasons. Once someone steps into this stage it is diffi-cult to turn back, and they continue along this line for months. After a period of time, the second stage occurs where the individual becomes used to this lifestyle, to feeling hungry, and to being depleted of various nutrients. The third stage occurs when the body itself responds to these changes, such as with a decrease in blood pressure, a drop in various hormone levels, and structural changes within the brain (Brumberg 2000).

BIOMEDICAL THEORY

Although Simmonds' disease and other endocrine models fell out of favor in the 1930s, new theories linking endocrine and neurologic abnormalities with anorexia have recently come back into play. These two systems have intrigued researchers in recent years because many of the signs and symptoms anorexics develop are regulated by hormones in the brain, including weight, balance, hunger, and satiety (fullness), blood pressure, development or regression of sex hormones, and menstruation. Scientists have proposed multiple theories in their search for the development of anorexia. The theories have ranged from hormone imbalances to abnormal functioning of the satiety center of the hypothalamus (the area of the brain that detects when someone is no longer hungry) to the role of stress in causing abnormal changes in the hypothalamus.

Results of studies completed over the last several years have provided evidence that there indeed may be one or more underlying biochemical abnormalities within the brain which predisposes some people to develop anorexia. Studies have indicated that when anorexics restrict their food intake, the levels of certain chemicals in the brain may change in an abnormal way. For example, dieting and food restriction have been shown, in some people, to cause a rise in the levels of endorphins and other chemicals, thereby leading to a feeling of accomplishment. Simultaneously, it has been shown to decrease the level of anxiety in these individuals. These two responses, which are the opposite of what would be expected in the typical individual, could provide an incentive for weight loss in those who respond abnormally. Researchers also postulate that prolonged starvation could cause chronic biochemical changes, such as a decrease in endorphin levels, when the individual eats. The drop in endorphin levels that goes along with eating would have the unfortunate effect of making the starved individual feel sad, so there is no incentive to eat (Frank et al. 2004).

There has been debate as to whether individuals with anorexia control their hunger or actually are not as hungry as those without anorexia. Newer research, which includes biochemical abnormalities, provides evidence that anorexics may actually not be as hungry or have the same desire to eat as those without an eating disorder. In addition, they may have earlier satiety. Studies have shown that they have an increased autonomic response to food, that looking at pictures of food causes feelings of fear and disgust in them, and that their response to appetite stimulants is not as intense. Highly caloric food, in particular, led to greater brain activity in anorexics than in the normal weight study group. Furthermore, body image distortions and food increase activity in specific regions of the brain, which remain activated after recovery. This information suggests that the specific areas of brain activation may have been different even before the onset of anorexia, leading to a greater risk of developing anorexia in these individuals (Frank et al. 2004).

Currently, research is being conducted on the role of several hormones in the development and treatment of anorexia, including ghrelin, leptin, and melanocortin. Several studies have shown potential benefits of administering ghrelin, a peptide produced mainly in the stomach that is related to and increases the effects of growth hormone. Administering ghrelin to patients with some medical illnesses has led to an increase in their appetites, resulting in weight gain. Naturally, scientists hoped that it would also stimulate the appetite in patients with anorexia nervosa but, to date, they have not been successful (Miljic et al. 2006). A second hormone being studied is leptin, which is produced mainly in fat cells and interacts with the hypothalamus to help regulate appetite and body weight. Normally, high leptin levels send a message to the brain that the body has had enough to eat. In fact, researchers documented that giving leptin to both thin and obese mice led to anorexia and loss of body fat (Kaibara et al. 1998). Contrary to normal controls, studies have shown that leptin levels may be inappropriately low in anorexics, thereby sending a premature message that the body has had enough to eat. Researchers contemplate whether this could potentially lead to anorexia. Therefore, to stimulate the appetite, there may be a potential benefit to inhibiting leptin in those with eating disorders. Melanocortin is also being considered as a hormone that may have a role in both the cause of and medical treatment for anorexia. Studies in mice have shown that inhibiting the receptor of melanocortin stimulates the appetite. Therefore, excess melanocortin may lead to anorexia and, conversely, inhibiting levels in anorexic patients may stimulate appetite.

Researchers have also been able to look at the brain and changes in brain activity through special imaging techniques, such as magnetic resonance spectroscopy and positron emission tomography. Their results have provided support for the theory that both hormones and the brain are involved in the development or maintenance of anorexia. Through these studies, researchers have found that many individuals with anorexia and bulimia have abnormal anatomy and activity within specific regions of the brain. Even after an anorexic recovers, these specific regions remain abnormal (W.H. Kaye et al. 2005). For example, the size of ventricles and volume of both gray and white matter within specific areas of the brain are decreased in anorexics. After recovery, only some of this volume loss resolves. Further research indicates that some of the abnormal activity in the brain may be due to a hormone within the brain, serotonin. Serotonin levels have been shown to be abnormal in individuals with eating disorders and persist after recovery. Researchers think that serotonin activity may be responsible for the anxiety, obsessive behavior, inhibition, and body image distortions seen during and possibly prior to the onset of anorexia. Furthermore, abnormal levels of serotonin may cause atypical emotional responses and feelings of reward, especially in response to eating and appetite. As with endorphins, the lack of eating may lead to an improved mood and lower anxiety levels, whereas eating may cause the opposite effect. Possible situations where an individual may have a rise in the level of serotonin and become a set up for the subsequent development of anorexia include the increase in sex hormone levels during puberty, stress, and cultural pressures which increase anxiety and, therefore, serotonin (W. Kaye 2008).

GENE THEORY

Family, twin, and adoption studies are all used to search for a genetic link to an illness. Indeed, studies performed on anorexics and their families have shown that heredity is a factor in the development of anorexia nervosa. In other words, some individuals may carry genes which make them more likely to develop anorexia than those without. Family studies are conducted to see whether certain families have more relatives with a specific disorder than other families. Although these studies provide valuable information, they can't definitively differentiate between a genetic, environmental, or social basis for the increased incidence within a family. Twin studies are very helpful in determining whether there is a genetic link to an illness because, while all siblings have similar environmental influences, identical twins have identical genetic material whereas fraternal twins don't. Therefore, if there is a genetic factor, identical twins should have a higher incidence of a genetic disorder than fraternal twins. Finally, adoption studies compare a child reared in a different environment from a sibling living in the original home. If there is a genetic link, then the risk of the adopted child developing an illness should be similar to or approach that of the other child. Results of all of these different types of studies show that anorexia is more common in certain families and that genetics does play a role. A large family study done in 2000 demonstrated that the risk for anorexia in female relatives of an affected individual was over 11 times higher than that for control subjects (Strober et al. 2000). Additionally, twin studies have shown that the risk of identical twins developing anorexia was much greater than that of fraternal twins, with heritability about 70%. Personality characteristics, symptoms, and behaviors that are associated with disordered eating have also been shown to be greater between identical than fraternal twins (Treasure, Schmidt, and Van Furth 2003). In 2002, researchers found that relatives of patients with eating disorders were more likely to exhibit characteristics of anorexics, such as perfectionism and being distrustful of others. Researchers have begun to evaluate the human genome and have found a possible genetic site responsible for the development of eating disorders (Tozzi, Bergen, and Bulik 2002). Further studies need to be conducted to verify these and to further evaluate the role of inheritance.

MULTIFACTORIAL THEORY

A newer, well-received theory is the multifactorial theory, where it is believed that risk factors add up to cause anorexia in susceptible individuals. Researchers think that individuals who are genetically susceptible to developing anorexia who are then exposed to a combination of chronic behavioral, biological, emotional, interpersonal, cultural, and social factors, are most likely to become ill. This model takes into account and includes aspects of other theories from the past few decades. Psychological factors which can increase the risk of an eating disorder include low self-esteem, a feeling of inadequacy or lack of control, depression, anxiety, anger, and loneliness. Interpersonal factors include problems expressing emotions and feelings, being teased about one's weight, or a history of physical or sexual abuse. They also include interactions within the family and a family's excessive focus on thinness, dieting, and extreme exercise. Sociocultural factors that contribute to the development of anorexia may include the cultural pressure to value or emulate those who are thin and beautiful. Multiple factors can add up and reinforce each other in individuals who are vulnerable, possibly because of a genetic predisposition or a certain biochemical profile. According to the multifactorial theory, susceptible individuals with multiple risk factors who decide to diet are the ones who develop anorexia nervosa, while those with similar influences and societal pressures but without the genetic or biochemical profile do not become ill.

7

Treatment of Anorexia Nervosa

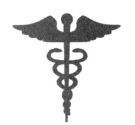

Life is simple as my parents' robot
I am determined to overachieve
I seem happy to accomplish a lot
Exhausted, I only rest when I heave
Eyes probe me while doctors divulge their find
Suffering spreads when I'm opened with knives
The truth seeps from my past, unconscious mind
Change is excruciating in our lives
Attempting to please others is all done
Depression appears as I recover
My own desires develop for fun
My contents emerge to be discovered
Happiness comes because of my freedom
I am myself ends this impassioned hum

—Ari

The eating disorders field is growing and therapists have more experience in working with anorexics than previously. Subsequently, they have developed a track record of success and failure (see Table 7.1).

Table 7.1

Treatment Recommendations for Patients who are Starving Themselves (1800s) or Diagnosed with Anorexia Nervosa

Time Period	Treatment
1870s	good food and nursing
	removal from the home environment, family, and friends
	diet of cream, milk, soup, eggs, fish and chicken to be given in two-hour intervals
	Heavy clothing along with "warm bed rest" and external heat on the spine, warm baths, massages
	Cooking favorite and desirable foods, electric shock, and forced bed rest
	Asylums for those who had nowhere else to go; intimidation and force feeding
1880s	insane asylum to teach proper moral behavior and for force feeding
1914–1930s	multiple hormone treatments, such as thyroid, growth hormone, insulin, antuitrin, and estrogen
1940s	Psychoanalysis
1970s	Family therapy
	Inpatient therapy on general hospital unit or psychiatric wards
1980s	Inpatient programs within special eating disorders units, private residential facilities
	Development of treatment team
1990s	Further development and specialization of treatment teams, including nutritionist, group therapist,
	Development of multiple family day programs and partial hospitalizations psychologist, psychiatrist
2000s	Development of Maudsley method
	Specialization of treatment based on specific patient characteristics, such as age and length of illness
	Medication trials (mostly in research)

In addition, researchers have analyzed theoretical models of anorexia and the outcomes of many treatment regimens. These two groups of specialists, researchers and therapists, now collaborate at national meetings to discuss different aspects of anorexia. They also read about different perspectives through the peer-reviewed journal, *The International Journal of Eating Disorders*. Many national organizations have developed extensive networks not only to raise money for research, but also to educate and support patients, families, and the public about anorexia. The massive amount of information that has been collected and analyzed has led to new ways of thinking about anorexia nervosa and new treatment plans. Despite all the time and effort, however, anorexia is still a very difficult illness to treat, and there is no consensus on the best plan. The long-term success rate is inadequate, where fewer than half of anorexics ever have a complete resolution of their illness, with many suffering relapses or eventually developing bulimia nervosa (Berkman et al. 2006). Unfortunately, anorexia still has the highest mortality rate of any mental illness.

A REVIEW OF CURRENT THERAPIES FOR ANOREXIA

A large, important study completed by the Agency for Health Research and Quality (AHRQ) in 2006 evaluated treatments for anorexia beginning in 1980. It assessed several types of psychotherapy used to treat anorexia, including cognitive, supportive, dynamic, family, individual, and group therapy. It also evaluated medications, including hormone treatments, tricyclic antidepressants, and fluoxetine, a newer antidepressant and anti-anxiety medicine (also known as a selective serotonin reuptake inhibitor). Successful outcomes were determined by the amount of weight the patient gained, in addition to the patient's actual weight at the end of treatment. Measures of psychological well-being were also evaluated, such as body dissatisfaction, the desire to be thin, return of menstruation, decrease in overall exercise, and the discontinuation of binging and purging.

Results of the AHRQ study show that in very few cases was one treatment found to be more successful than another, and no treatment was highly effective in treating all cases of anorexia. They did have some positive results, however. First, they determined that adolescents newly diagnosed with anorexia did relatively well with individual therapy. In fact, young teens who were ill for only a short period of time did better than any other age group. Second, adults with a long history of anorexia were less likely to relapse if they reached a normal weight while undergoing cognitive behavioral therapy. Third, they found that family therapy, which focuses on teaching parents how to control the nutritional aspect of the illness, was helpful for younger adolescents but not for adults. The other part of the study which evaluated medications found that they did not help patients gain weight. If, however, a patient had a co-morbid diagnosis, such as depression, it helped resolve these symptoms (Berkman et al. 2006).

Results from studies such as this, along with physicians' clinical experiences, have led researchers and therapists to conclude that a treatment plan with multiple components is better than therapy alone, and that it often needs to be individualized. The specific type of therapy one ultimately chooses depends on a variety of factors, including their age, comfort level, strengths, weaknesses, living situation, and severity of the illness. Unfortunately, financial ability and type of health insurance are also major components in determining a treatment plan. All of these factors will not only determine what type of therapy might be best for the patient, but also the best place for the patient to receive treatment, which can vary from going to scheduled outpatient appointments to being an inpatient in an eating disorders center.

THE RELATIONSHIP BETWEEN A THERAPIST AND ANOREXIC

No matter what type of therapy an anorexic receives, a good relationship between the patient and therapist is necessary for treatment to be successful. The initial encounter can be adversarial because anorexics are usually satisfied with their current lifestyle and don't want to enter therapy. Instead, they are pressured by a parent, husband, physician, or college, which may require students with eating disorders to see a counselor and maintain a certain weight to attend classes. The therapist's first job is to convince anorexics that they personally want to work on issues that led to the weight loss and abnormal behaviors. Therapists are aware that there are a series of stages that people must undergo before they decide to make a behavioral change, whether it is eating more, quitting smoking, or leaving an abusive relationship. Anorexics usually enter therapy in the first stage, where they have no desire to change their weight or eating habits. Therapists encourage and guide them through each successive stage, which progresses from *considering* to change an undesirable behavior, to *deciding* that they want to change, to *taking specific steps* to change the behavior and, finally, *incorporating* the new, healthier behavior into their lives.

Besides motivating the anorexic to want to change, the therapist also focuses on building a positive, trusting relationship so the anorexic feels comfortable exploring experiences which led to the current problems. In fact, the patient often learns to depend on the therapist greatly during therapy. This type of bond, called a therapeutic alliance, is important for anybody who enters therapy, but is particularly significant for anorexics for two reasons. First, many have not been able to trust or depend on adult role models in the past so trusting an adult authority figure in therapy can be very difficult. Second, the therapist is asking anorexics to explore every aspect of their current lives and change much of what they have built to protect themselves.

Treating someone with anorexia can be extremely challenging, and not all therapists feel comfortable working with them. As mentioned previously, anorexics are reluctant to change. Because of this, they can be rigid, secretive, and manipulative, making it difficult to treat them or follow their progress.

For instance, anorexics commonly place weights in their clothes or drink a lot of water immediately before their scheduled weight checks so it appears they weigh more than they actually do. In addition, they often hide the fact that a certain topic is personally relevant to their situation, so a therapist has difficulty deciding which specific topics to explore with them. Furthermore, some therapists fear that what they say or do in therapy could have a negative effect and cause further weight loss and, perhaps, the need to be hospitalized. Plus, those who are dangerously thin may repeatedly require hospitalization, causing long gaps and interruptions in therapy (Levenkron 2000).

CHOOSING THE RIGHT TYPE OF THERAPY

There are literally hundreds of types of therapies for someone with a psychological issue, but the major types used with anorexics are interpersonal, cognitive-behavioral, and family therapy. Newer models which combine various aspects of these have also been developed. In addition, therapists sometimes tailor a treatment to fit an individual's needs. Sometimes one particular therapy will be recommended over another, or the parents or individual with anorexia will feel more comfortable with a certain philosophy. It is important to remember, however, that no matter what type of therapy is chosen, the chances of a successful outcome increase when two conditions are fulfilled. First, the patient must be ready to make changes. Fortunately, the initial stage of most therapeutic approaches deals with this issue. Second, the individual must be above a certain target weight before therapy can be effective because the state of extreme starvation leads to rigid and abnormal thought processes.

PSYCHOANALYSIS

One of the oldest types of psychotherapy is psychoanalysis. Psychoanalysis was developed by Sigmund Freud and is often seen in an exaggerated form in movies, where the patient is on a couch while the therapist sits on a chair with a notepad. In order for patients to successfully participate in psychoanalysis, they must be motivated, relatively healthy, and prepared for a long time commitment. Typically, sessions occur four to five times a week for several years. True psychoanalysis is not used as often today as it was years ago. First, it is time-consuming and, second, anorexics are usually unable to remain actively engaged for such an extended period of time. After this period of active involvement, the therapy loses its effectiveness and behaviors that have not been successfully dealt with are more likely to become a permanent part of the patient's lifestyle.

PSYCHODYNAMIC AND INTERPERSONAL THERAPY

Two other types of psychotherapy currently used with anorexics are psychodynamic and interpersonal therapy. The theory behind psychodynamic therapy is that people are able to identify the psychological and interpersonal factors in their personal history which led to their current behaviors. Once they have figured out the reason for their actions and behaviors, they are then able to make changes.

Another type of psychotherapy, called interpersonal therapy, was first used as a relatively short-term treatment for patients with depression. Later, this treatment was generalized to other mental illnesses, including anorexia. In fact, it has been shown to be the most effective therapy for anorexics that are young, received their diagnosis less than three years before, are stable, and highly motivated. The goal of interpersonal therapy is to identify what caused the onset and persistence of the anorexia in the patient's personal history, looking specifically at relationships and conflicts with others. For example, there may be an issue within the family, such as a lack of warmth or communication, unrealistic expectations, or sexual abuse. The therapist helps the patient uncover these issues to work through them and, simultaneously, attempts to increase the patient's independence and self-esteem. Interpersonal therapy concentrates on current issues and conflicts rather than on specific behaviors and symptoms. If a patient complains of a certain issue, the therapist will work with the patient to try to identify why the specific behavior emerged, rather than discuss the issue itself.

As with other treatments, there are three distinct treatment components to interpersonal therapy, and the patient must participate in all stages to successfully complete therapy. The first stage is to discover the problems that may have led to the weight loss. The second is to work on the problem areas, and the third stage is to put all the separate pieces together and come up with a plan to work in the "real" world. During the first stage of therapy, the therapist discusses what it means to have anorexia nervosa, what the symptoms are, and the treatment. The therapist asks many questions to try to determine what relationship difficulties or life experiences may have led to the patient's problems. These events and how they could have influenced the patient become the major focus of the rest of therapy. The therapist helps by recognizing repetitive patterns that occur within relationships, discovering events that may be responsible for the onset and maintenance of anorexia, and helping to devise a list of goals for the patient. Since interpersonal therapy is supposed to be short-term, it is one of few therapies that operates on a deadline, rather than letting patients work at their own pace.

COGNITIVE-BEHAVIORAL THERAPY

Cognitive-behavioral therapy (CBT) is also a time-limited therapy which has been shown to prevent relapses in some adults with chronic anorexia. Unfortunately, many chronic anorexics who gain weight during this treatment will still eventually lose weight again. As the name indicates, there are two parts to this type of therapy. The first is the educational aspect, where the therapist teaches the patient about the characteristics of anorexia. Aaron Beck (1921–), a psychiatrist who developed a cognitive model of therapy in the 1960s and 1970s, believes that emotional disorders are influenced by unpleasant thoughts, and particular behaviors are due to a distorted interpretation of facts. The idea is that an anorexic can be taught to use objective data, such as a scale or book with normal weight for height values to correctly interpret facts. For example, one goal is to differentiate between the thought, "I am fat;" the feeling, "I feel fat;" and the reality, "I am significantly underweight." Beck also believes that patients with emotional disorders develop an all-or-nothing way of thinking about things, such as "I am fat" or "I am thin." Although Beck mainly used his theories to explain a depressive disorder, other therapists, including David Garner and Kelly Bemis-Vitousek, adapted and applied them to anorexics. They have theorized that those who have anorexia believe that "thin" is good, whereas "not thin" is bad, worthless, and imperfect. Their behavior is to do whatever is possible to become thin and, therefore, good, worthy, and perfect. Self-worth becomes defined by body weight and shape.

The second aspect of CBT is behavioral. After the therapist and anorexic have discovered the distorted thoughts and beliefs, they then work on the behaviors which developed as a result of these beliefs. Together, the therapist and patient identify new, more appropriate behaviors which the patient then goes out and tests. During this phase of treatment, the patient also writes in a home journal daily to improve the chances that she or he will discover other distorted thoughts and abnormal behaviors. Proponents of this theory believe that, while the patient is the one exhibiting the dangerous behaviors, others help to perpetuate or maintain the weight loss efforts through positive reinforcement. For example, anorexics may begin to lose weight because it makes them feel better, less anxious, and in greater control. Friends and families, however, reinforce and provide further support for their weight loss goals when they tell them how good they look and pay more attention to them than they had previously.

FAMILY THERAPY

Maria Selvini Palazzoli was one of the first major contributors to the family therapy model. This type of therapy has been shown to be more helpful for younger patients, especially those who have had anorexia for less than three years. Even young patients who are severely affected may be able to stay in the home if their parents are actively involved and receive help and guidance through family therapy. In the late 1970s, the first study which evaluated the effectiveness of family therapy reported that 86% of the patients had recovered at the time of the study. Their patient sample consisted mainly of young adolescents who had been diagnosed with anorexia an average of slightly over 18 months before treatment began (Minuchin, Rosman, and Baker 1978). Other studies have shown that benefits continued years after therapy. More recent studies in teens have shown that one-half to two-thirds will be a healthy weight at the end of therapy and, at follow up, 60% to 90% will have recovered while 10% to 15% will remain sick (Treasure, Schmidt, and Van Furth 2003). Although there has been some success with young adults, it has not been nearly as good as those seen with the younger patient group, who continue to have recovery rates much higher than any other group of anorexics.

Currently, successful family therapy doesn't concentrate on relationship problems within the family, but instead focuses on teaching members of the family how to help the affected child. One particular aspect of family therapy that has shown to be particularly useful is teaching a parent how to be an active member in the recovery process and how to take control of their child's reintroduction to food. For example, parents can help plan daily meals and snacks, prepare food to be eaten together as a family, shop for specific foods, and provide positive, objective support and encouragement. Another important aspect of family therapy is teaching parents how to reintroduce their child into family life and not to separate the child from family activities which are not directly related to the anorexia. In addition, parents are taught to control their own anxieties and fears regarding their child and to take control of their child's illness. They also learn how to externalize the anorexia so that the illness becomes the problem to deal with and does not define the entire familial relationship.

Family therapy has been helpful for many adolescents and aspects of it continue to be used today. Despite some success with the actual treatment, specialists do not agree with the original theory that led to the therapy. When the family model was originally developed, Selvini Palazzoli, Bruch, and other therapists believed that the patient became ill because the family relationship was dysfunctional. This type of family was labeled the "psychosomatic family," and the initial goal of therapy was to teach the family to interact in a more positive way. Recent research does not support the theory that anorexia is caused solely by dysfunctional families and, in fact, has demonstrated that families of anorexics are diverse in their interactions and responses to one another, their emotional characteristics, and their sociocultural environment.

More recently, variations of the family therapy model, which are not based on the psychosomatic family, have been developed and can be useful for families who need help and support. For example, if the parents of an anorexic are having a marital problem which is impacting the child, therapy may be recommended. Alternatively, if the child lives in a single parent household, the parent may need extra help and guidance on how to work effectively with the child. In addition, if the anorexic is married, both partners may need to attend couple's therapy to discuss how the illness is affecting the relationship, marriage, and children. Issues such as trust, dependency, parenting, and the ability to act in a supportive manner are all discussed.

MAUDSLEY METHOD

A relatively new type of treatment for anorexia is the Maudsley method, a treatment developed by Christopher Dare and Ivan Eisler at Maudsley Hospital in London. To date, studies have shown encouraging results in younger adolescents but not in other patient groups. The Maudsley method draws from the most successful aspects of other programs. Mainly, parents assume the responsibility for making sure their adolescent eats. Dare and Eisler believe that, in most cases, the family is not dysfunctional and, therefore, should not be blamed for either the onset or maintenance of anorexia in their child. In essence, the anorexic should be treated as if the illness is medical rather than psychological, and the parents should nurse their child back to health (Dare et al. 2000). In this medical illness model, food is identical to medicine and the parents are cast as healers.

The treatment, like others, is broken into three stages. The first is the weight restoration stage. Parents learn how to encourage and take responsibility for their child's eating. They learn strategies to convince the anorexic to eat, to enforce rules related to eating, and to effectively deal with anxiety surrounding food. Parents are allowed to provide incentives to coax their child to eat. Although the therapist is available to provide support, reassurance, and encouragement during this initial, difficult phase there is not direct intervention. Anorexics are encouraged to turn to siblings and peers to receive support because it will help them form more age and developmentally appropriate bonds and relationships. The second stage of therapy begins when the anorexic agrees to follow the rules related to eating and is consistently gaining weight. During this stage, parents help their child assume more responsibility for and control over their eating. Once the anorexic has reached and maintained 95% of the ideal body weight with minimal help from others, the third phase of treatment begins. During this stage, outpatient therapy is initiated to help the adolescent develop a healthy adolescent identity. Therapy also allows teens to examine issues and anxieties regarding adolescence and to learn how to set boundaries for themselves and others. One problem with the Maudsley method is that it requires a major time commitment from the family. Parents must supervise meals, deal with food refusal, and consistently enforce food-related rules. In addition, they need to be able to separate themselves from the interpersonal issues that have dominated the family throughout the illness (Le Grange and Lock n.d.).

Ari distinctly recalls going through these stages with her family. She remembers when she began to eat again. "My new meal requirements addressed every fear of my anorexia nervosa. I placed myself in solitary to cut the new foods into miniscule pieces. My mom prepared my exact meals for me and I was terrified that she was slipping pure fat into my food." She also recalls the support she received from her family.

> My family carried me through these tough times. They sat with me, held me, and rocked me during my toughest breakdowns. My mom analyzed my previous actions with me and was always by my side ... My dad rationally reviewed my life with me and helped me ... My brother would try to make me laugh, and he would bring a glimmer of a smile to my anguished face. Every time I had a good day or accomplished a small chore, my sister would have me run through streamers and break through the finish line.

SPECIALIST SUPPORTIVE CLINICAL MANAGEMENT

Specialist supportive clinical management (SSCM) is another new and promising therapeutic model that also draws from established and effective treatments, including basic clinical management and supportive psychotherapy. Initial results based on a small number of trials have shown improved outcome over several other types of therapy. One advantage to this treatment plan is that it is relatively easy to implement compared to some of the others. The clinical management aspect emphasizes educating the patient about important features of anorexia through verbal and written information. Sample topics include signs and symptoms of anorexia and warning signs of a recurrence. SSCM also requires regular monitoring and follow-up with a health care provider, including lab tests, weight measurements, electrocardiograms, and other objective health measurements. The supportive psychotherapy piece of the model uses support, affection, reassurance, and hope to develop a positive alliance between the therapist and patient in working toward a common goal.

The therapist emphasizes strengths, provides praise, and acts as an attentive listener who uses a conversational style when speaking, asking open-ended questions and reflecting on past comments or events. This type of therapy is much more flexible than others, as the patient can bring up issues at each session which may or may not carry over to the next. SSCM has three stages of therapy, the first of which is a discussion of SSCM and the identification of agreed-on target symptoms and goals. The second stage consists mainly of monitoring, support, and encouragement. The final phase is a review of issues, finalizing therapy, and developing goals and plans for the future.

GROUP THERAPY

Group therapy is used as an adjunct to individual therapy, especially at colleges and universities. In addition, groups can form in inpatient and outpatient treatment centers. Patients like it because it makes them feel less lonely, and it allows them to share their thoughts and feelings with others who can empathize. However, therapists have learned that group therapy is risky because younger patients can learn new ways of losing weight, purging, or manipulating others by listening to older, more experienced group members. Therefore, facilitators make every effort possible to form a group which includes anorexics that are around the same age and illness level.

NUTRITIONAL THERAPY

In addition to therapists, other professionals play an important role in the treatment of anorexics, particularly nutritionists. Nutritionists who work with anorexics must understand the intense fear they have surrounding food and weight gain. In general, these specialists educate their patients about food and calories. Initially, they provide structured meal plans for the anorexics to follow. They also teach them about daily requirements, how many calories they need to maintain their current weight, and the number of calories needed to gain enough weight to reach a target goal. Nutritionists work with the patient's therapist to devise a weight gain plan. At first the gain is slow and at an agreed-on rate, but the eventual goal set by the treatment team is a weight gain of one-half to two pounds per week. Anorexics usually begin with a meal plan that totals about 1,000 to 2,000 calories each day (Fisher 2006). As the body becomes accustomed to more food, the number of calories consumed each day is slowly increased by 200 to 400 until the anorexic is eating about 2,000 to 3,000 calories per day. As a point of reference, the average adult male and female usually consume around 2,500 and 2,000 calories a day, respectively.

Sometimes an anorexic who is trying to gain weight may need to eat twice as much as someone who is maintaining their current weight (APA Steering Committee on Practice Guidelines 2006). If an anorexic is not gaining enough weight because of inadequate intake, the team of professionals working with the patient will provide a target weight, and if this number cannot be reached or maintained, then the patient will be hospitalized.

Ari remembers when she began to eat again and how difficult and slow it was at first.

My entire body tightened and each limb locked in place, supporting the determination of my mind. I slowly, painfully put a tiny, cut-up piece of meat into my mouth. It only took one slight chew and a forced swallow to finish the first bite of a meal that would take hours to complete. That small piece of meat crept down my throat, down my chest, all the way to my stomach and I would feel the weight of the food and the expectancy of the rest of the meal. This is the fight that I battled every second of my recovery.

Nutritionists also help to plan and choose menus, teaching patients how to select appropriate food choices and, over time, allow them to plan their own menus. They encourage anorexics to choose a variety of food choices and evaluate their selections. In addition, they monitor weight gain progress by a variety of measurements, including skin fold thickness, percent body fat, weight for height, and BMI. Nutritionists recommend appropriate dietary supplements based on the patient's weight, diet, and levels of specific nutrients, such as iron and calcium.

SELF-HELP GROUPS

In addition to professional services, many self-help groups were formed in the 1970s when families became concerned and frustrated because they either could not find a therapist who was willing to treat their family member, or the therapist they found did not know much about anorexia. Some of the first self-help groups were Eating Disorders Awareness and Prevention Inc., the American Anorexia Bulimia Association (these two groups merged to form the National Eating Disorders Association), and the National Association of Anorexia Nervosa and Associated Disorders (ANAD) (Gordon 2000). With the advent of the Internet, these organizations are often the first resource people use when they think that they or a family member may have a problem. The organizations provide education, support, resource information, and recommendations. Some offer chat rooms, where one can share feelings and concerns with others who have or had anorexia or, alternatively, with professionals who specialize in eating disorders.

MAJOR TREATMENT SETTINGS

Whereas it is clear that anorexics need to receive therapy, families need to choose not only the specific type of therapy but also the best place for the anorexic to receive it. The National Eating Disorders Association (NEDA) has published general guidelines and treatment recommendations based on the severity of the illness. The options range from outpatient treatment to partial hospitalization to inpatient or residential treatment settings.

Outpatient Treatment

When someone has been diagnosed with anorexia but is medically and psychiatrically stable, a therapist will most likely recommend outpatient treatment. A typical candidate for this type of treatment is someone who is young and newly diagnosed, who may intermittently meet all the criteria for the diagnosis, and who has never required hospitalization. Outpatient treatment usually consists of more than one type of service, and can include nutritional counseling, psychological counseling, and medical follow-up. If the patient has an additional or co-morbid diagnosis, such as depression or anxiety, a psychiatrist or other medical doctor will need to prescribe medication. Counseling may be offered by a psychiatrist, a licensed psychologist, a social worker, or other types of counselors. A *psychiatrist* is a medical doctor (M.D.) who specializes in psychiatry and is the only type of therapist who can prescribe medications and provide true psychoanalysis. A *psychologist* has a doctorate degree (Ph.D. or PsyD.) who has received several years of training and clinical experience beyond undergraduate school. A *licensed clinical social worker* (LCSW) has a master's degree in social work and has specialized in guiding clients to improve their lives. Other therapists who work with anorexics and families of anorexics include *marriage or family therapists, licensed professional counselors,* and *pastoral counselors.*

Outpatient Day Programs and Partial Hospitalization

There are a variety of programs available for patients who need more structure or guidance than they can receive by attending therapy sessions once or twice a week. Outpatient day programs and partial hospitalization programs were developed for two specific groups of anorexics who need extra services. The first group includes anorexics who are not improving adequately with outpatient therapy, but who aren't sick enough to be admitted into an inpatient setting. The second group includes anorexics that have just been discharged from an inpatient setting but are not yet ready to resume their old lives. Depending on the outpatient day program, anorexics usually attend anywhere from three to eight hours a day, although not every day of the week. Usually, those who attend these programs also continue to go to work or school. Partial hospitalization programs, viewed as a treatment for those who have just been released from the hospital, often have their patients attend for at least six hours daily.

Although there are many similarities among the programs in the United States and Europe, there is no standard treatment. This is demonstrated in a study done in 2002, where researchers reviewed the types of services offered to anorexics within twelve European countries. They found that all countries offered outpatient, day, and inpatient programs, and all stressed the importance of mealtime and eating together. However, they also noted several differences between the programs, including the length of the program and services provided. For example, the number of days patients attended each week varied between one and four, and the length of treatment ranged from 10 to 36 weeks. In addition, services and activities provided, such as body image therapy, tennis, drama and field trips, varied by center (Gowers et al. 2002).

One well-known type of day program, called the multiple family therapy day program (MFDT), has been offered in both Dresden, Germany and London, England since the late 1990s. The two programs are similar in that they offer a variety of services, including intensive treatment for anorexics and their families, while attempting to keep the anorexics in their own homes. One difference between the programs is that the London unit is more rigid with respect to their daily schedule. Otherwise, both have a multidisciplinary team which includes nurses, psychologists, psychiatrists, occupational therapists, social workers, nutritionists, and teachers. Both programs also stress and intensively work with anorexics to reduce their social isolation and improve their relationships with others. The therapists also work intensively with families. For example, they teach families how to take an active role in the anorexic's recovery. Therapists also work with families to help them understand how the anorexic has changed the entire family's life and the family's relationship with others. By providing insight into these abnormal relationships, therapists are then able to help relatives make changes toward a more normal family life. In addition, group therapists provide opportunities for families and patients to meet and identify with others in a similar situation, where they are sometimes encouraged to participate in activities, such as role playing and art therapy.

INPATIENT TREATMENT

In the early 1970s, patients with life-threatening anorexia were placed in a general medical unit or psychiatric ward within a hospital because special eating disorder units in public and private hospitals didn't exist. Staff did not have the expertise to deal with these patients, who were often secretive, manipulative, and self-absorbed. As a result, the nurses often became quite frustrated and thought anorexics were spoiled brats because, unlike other patients, they appeared to be normal teens who refused to eat to the point of making themselves dangerously thin. Since the staff was not trained to work with anorexics, they often resorted to bullying and forced them to eat.

Over the next decade, private hospitals and specialized units within hospitals were developed and the medical personnel learned to work better with anorexics. Today, nurses are a very important part of an anorexic's hospitalization because they spend more time with the patient than any other health provider and are the main enforcers of rules and medical orders. Nurses are trained to be firm but sensitive and, instead of developing an antagonistic relationship, they learn how to become an important part of the patient's support system. In addition to nurses, physicians are also an important part of the health team. In fact, the team leader in an inpatient setting is often a psychiatrist, who manages the overall care. This provider makes the initial diagnosis, along with any additional co-morbid diagnoses, orders necessary tests, manages medical problems due to malnutrition, and orders medications. Sometimes, the team leader is a psychologist, who can also make the initial diagnosis or diagnoses and provide therapy. Other professionals on the team may include a family therapist and nutritionist.

These days, health care providers try to keep anorexics out of the hospital and managed at home. Although most can be treated on an outpatient basis or in day treatment programs, some still need to be hospitalized because they are medically or psychologically unstable. There are specific reasons that an anorexic needs to be placed in a hospital setting. These include:

- Less than 75% ideal body weight or continued weight loss despite treatment
- Refusal to eat
- Body fat less than 10%
- Heart rate less than 50 beats per minute during the day and less than 45 beats per minute at night
- Systolic blood pressure less than 90 mm Hg

- Orthostatic changes in the pulse (changes when one lies down and then stands up) of over 20 beats per minute or blood pressure of over 10 mm Hg
- Core body temperature less than 96 degrees F (35.6 degrees C)
- An arrhythmia, or abnormal heart beat
- Suicide plan or attempt

The reason these criteria were chosen is because, in these situations, the anorexic's body often begins to shut down, significantly increasing the risk of a medical emergency or death. For example, when a heart rate is extremely low because of a decreased metabolism, the heart may not function normally and the patient is at significant risk of developing abnormal rhythms or heart failure. Similar heart problems can occur when the heart muscle mass shrinks due to muscle breakdown. In addition, a low blood pressure can keep blood from reaching important organs, so the organs will fail.

Once a family or patient decides that they need to be hospitalized for emergent care, they may choose a general hospital with a psychiatric or specialized eating disorder unit, or a private center which can handle medically ill anorexics. Unfortunately, anorexics who are admitted into hospitals spend much less time there today than they did 20 years ago. In the 1980s, anorexics who entered inpatient eating disorder programs stayed as long as they needed, even months at a time, because insurance companies did not set time limits. In 1984, the average inpatient stay in the United States was 149.5 days (Frisch, Herzog, and Franko 2006). Consequently, they were able to receive comprehensive care, including an adjustment period at the beginning of their hospitalization and extensive discharge planning. In 2006, the average time an anorexic spent in the hospital was 26 days, compared to 40.6 to 135.8 days in Europe (Bulik et al. 2007). This is because insurance companies in the United States have strict criteria regarding what, when, and how much they will reimburse for inpatient hospitalizations. Insurance companies use weight as the main criterion for discharge, whereas professionals also consider psychological well-being an important factor in determining when to discharge a patient. According to ANAD, a major reason for relapse is being discharged prematurely from a hospital because families can't afford to pay the cost of what insurance companies refuse to reimburse. Unfortunately, the cost of treating an anorexic in the hospital is very expensive and requires more time and money than insurance companies are willing to cover. According to data from the Agency for Health, Research and Quality, in 2003, an average 16½-day hospitalization for a patient with anorexia was approximately $30,970.

INPATIENT THERAPY CONCENTRATES ON WEIGHT GAIN

Anorexics admitted into a hospital setting receive traditional therapies along with more emergent treatments. The major goal for severely malnourished anorexics is to increase their weight. However, before that can be done, the treatment team must ensure that electrolyte levels and fluid balances are normal. Once this is done, nutritionists will work with the rest of the treatment team to come up with a feeding plan. The weight goal for an inpatient, two to three pounds per week, is greater than for an outpatient (Lucas 2004).

Anorexics who are hospitalized are often given the chance to continue to feed themselves and eat on their own. One model used to try to encourage them to eat and gain weight is behavior modification, a therapy which is based on reward and punishment. Basically, the patient is given a target weight gain which must be met. If the goal is met, the patient receives certain rewards or privileges, such as being able to watch television or have a more flexible daily schedule, particularly regarding eating. If the goal is not met, privileges are removed and the structure surrounding the day, especially meals, often becomes more rigid. Although it does not help the patient determine the reason for the anorexia or how to cope with it, it does increase food consumption and weight gain in the short-term so the anorexic can think more clearly and perform better in therapy.

Under extreme circumstances, if the anorexic refuses to eat, calories and nutrition must be given either through a nasogastric tube (NG tube) or through an intravenous line (IV). NG feeding involves providing liquid nutrition through a tube that goes from the nose into the stomach. IV nutrition involves placing an IV in the patient's vein and providing calories and nutrition through fluids, called "hyperalimentation" (Fisher 2006). Many professionals think that NG feeding is better than giving nutrition through an IV because there are fewer serious side effects. Also, NG feeds can be given at home. On the other hand, some experts prefer providing nutrition through an IV because they think it is less harmful psychologically and eliminates the feeling that others are torturing or overpowering the patient. Proponents of this method are concerned that force feeding the patient will damage the important therapeutic alliance or, in patients who have been sexually or physically abused, will associate the two events (Silber 2009).

No matter which method is chosen, refeeding must be done very carefully. Because of the anorexic's low metabolic state, it takes longer for food to leave the stomach and enter the small intestine. Any amount of food can cause problems such as severe stomach pains, diarrhea, and a feeling of fullness. Also, the increase in calories and energy provided by food suddenly increases the metabolic rate, causing symptoms such as a fast heart rate, sweating, and shortness of breath. Feeding too much and too quickly can cause the "refeeding syndrome," which is a sudden change in the levels of fluids and electrolytes within the body. Large amounts of carbohydrates can cause a sudden drop in the phosphate level, which may lead to sudden heart failure, seizures, coma, and death. Low phosphate levels can also cause vomiting, severe bone and joint pain, weakness, and loss of appetite. Furthermore, large amounts of salt, water, and protein, seen more often with IV nutrition, can overload the circulation and heart because of its poor functioning as a result of the loss of muscle mass. Less commonly, it can lead to a breakdown of the red blood cells, causing anemia and, therefore, decreased availability of oxygen for the body.

MEDICATIONS TO HELP WITH WEIGHT GAIN

Multiple studies have been conducted to to try to improve weight gain in anorexics through medications. To date, none have shown well-documented, significant improvement in weight gain or psychological well-being unless there is a co-morbid diagnosis. Antidepressants, such as fluoxetine, have helped resolve depression in anorexics, but haven't led to a significant weight change or normalization of body image issues. Other medications, such as cyproheptidine, have been used to try to stimulate the appetite, but without much success. Zinc supplementation has also been suggested to increase weight gain (Treasure, Schmidt, and Van Furth 2003). Since low zinc levels have reportedly caused changes in the levels of neurotransmitters within the brain similar to those seen with anorexics, and since many anorexics are deficient in several nutritional parameters, including zinc, researchers hypothesized that giving supplemental zinc might improve their abnormal parameters. Although few studies have been done to evaluate zinc supplementation, there has been limited success, necessitating further evaluation of this supplementation (Silber 2005). Cisapride, a medication which helps move food out of the stomach and into the intestines more quickly, decreased uncomfortable feelings of abdominal fullness but did not lead to improved weight gain. Researchers also hoped that olanzapine, an atypical antipsychotic, could potentially help with extreme symptoms of anorexia, such as the extreme fear of gaining weight, significant rituals, disordered thinking, and delusional body images. One of the medication's side effects, weight gain, was also a positive feature for anorexia treatment (Steffen et al. 2006). Although a few studies have shown potential benefits, to date there are not an adequate number of patients evaluated to know whether olanzapine is truly beneficial.

RESIDENTIAL TREATMENT CENTERS

Anorexics that have been ill for many years or have not had success in other programs may choose to attend a private, for-profit residential treatment program. The first private facility to treat anorexia, the Renfrew Center, opened in Philadelphia in 1985, and today there are many residential treatment centers which specialize in treating patients with eating disorders. Unfortunately, it is difficult to know which center will be beneficial because they are not regulated. Furthermore, there is no published information regarding their effectiveness or quality of care. Another drawback to these centers is their prohibitive expense. Insurance companies don't usually pay for residential centers that may charge $550 to $1,500 per day. The average length of stay is 83 days, making the total out of pocket expense over $79,000 (Frisch, Herzog, and Franko 2006).

There have been significant advances in the treatment of anorexia over the past several decades. Professionals are now more knowledgeable about how to work with rather than against anorexics, and specific models are being developed which are proving beneficial for specific patient groups, particularly those who are younger and newly diagnosed. Despite the advances, the risk of recurrence and chronic illness is still high, particularly for older patients. New methods need to be evaluated and implemented to improve the quality of life and cure rates in this group.

8

Prevention and Future Research

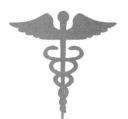

"I won't let myself look at magazines anymore because all I see are tiny, unreasonable people."

—Ari

RESEARCH IN PREVENTION

Time and experience has helped us gain a better understanding of anorexia nervosa, how to recognize it, diagnose it, and treat it. We know that making a diagnosis and beginning treatment early in the illness significantly increases the chance of recovery. Unfortunately, we don't have a clear understanding of how to prevent it, if this is indeed possible. Research in the field of anorexia prevention is new, and specialists are finding that the results are different than they had initially expected. For example, researchers thought techniques which worked to prevent other risky health behaviors would also work to help prevent anorexia. Often, teaching about dangers and risks associated with a specific behavior is enough to change people's attitudes and to reduce their likelihood of developing that risky behavior. Knowing this, researchers developed a model for anorexia prevention which is similar to that used for other undesirable health behaviors. Experts thought that teaching about the unrealistically thin female and society's obsession with the "thin ideal" would provide teens and young adults with some insight into their own thoughts about weight and starvation. The researchers believed that insight would be enough to change people's attitude and behavior. Unfortunately, this has not been the case with anorexia (Lucas 2004). Clinical studies have shown that educating children and teens about signs and symptoms of anorexia has not led to a decrease in the thoughts and behaviors that lead to anorexia. Contrarily, detailed information may actually provide adolescents with new incentives and methods to take control of their lives and make their lives seem less overwhelming. Anorexics who learn how to lose weight by watching, reading, or seeing how others do it are called "copycat anorexics" (Bruch 1978).

Other studies have also found that educating people about anorexia can have an undesirable effect. For example, recently researchers evaluated the impact of an eating disorders prevention program on a group of high school students. They divided the students into two groups, one whose presenter was an attractive "recovered anorexic," while the other was a "specialist" who never had anorexia. Although the researchers did see some positive effects on about half the students, they also discovered a disturbing response. More students in the group led by the "recovered anorexic" thought that girls with eating disorders were "pretty, in control of their lives, and could lead normal lives once they recovered," than girls who were led by the specialist. In addition, by the end of the program the first group of students viewed anorexics more positively than the second group. The researchers were concerned that students in the first group would be more likely to want to emulate the recovered anorexic after they completed the program than they would have been otherwise (Schwartz et al. 2007). Another study showed similar results. Educators taught an 8-week eating disorders prevention program, 45 minutes weekly, to 13- and 14-year-old schoolgirls. Although the girls were more knowledgeable and had fewer risky behaviors at the end of the program, by six months after completing the program, they were restricting their food intake more than at baseline (Carter et al. 1998).

PREVENTION AT HOME

Despite the disappointing results found regarding some prevention programs offered at school, there are things which can be done at home. Many self-help organizations and professional societies have made basic recommendations for families to help prevent their children from developing an eating disorder. A large amount of information is available on Web sites which are dedicated to preventing anorexia, and also to supporting families and patients with anorexia nervosa. The Anorexia Nervosa and Related Eating Disorders (ANDRED) Web site provides tips for parents. First, they stress how important it is to have a mother and/or another female authority figure, such as an aunt, act as a positive role model. Second, they emphasize that mothers should not criticize their own body or appearance, nor should they talk frequently about dieting. Instead, ANRED stresses that parents should emphasize proper nutrition and adequate exercise for themselves and their families. In addition, parents should discourage other family members from dieting, unless it is absolutely necessary. Furthermore, fathers should not criticize anyone else's appearance, especially that of his daughter or wife. This includes joking or calling relatives or others derogatory names which imply they are overweight or unattractive, such as "thunder thighs."

ANRED also stresses the importance of concentrating on healthy choices and emphasizes healthy bodies rather than thin ones. Parents can accomplish this by making mealtimes fun and easy going. In general, food should be varied and healthful. However, specific foods should not be forbidden but, instead, should be eaten in moderation. In addition, parents should role model how food can be enjoyable and fun for the entire family. In fact, families should make a point of eating out or having a special meal weekly. While it is fine to watch what one eats during these meals, it is important to remember that nobody should obsess over the amount of fat or number of calories they consume.

Parents also have an important role in educating their children about unrealistic cultural expectations. In fact, they must talk to their children about the unrealistic female ideal that is portrayed in all types of media, especially television and magazines. Not only do they need to talk about the dangerously thin models and actresses, but they should also discuss topics such as cosmetic surgery, airbrushing, computer manipulation, and other techniques used to enhance photos before they are placed in magazines. Similarly, parents should educate their children and teens about advertising, where the advertiser tries to entice the consumer to buy a certain product. Often, the model who is advertising the product is ridiculously thin. She convinces others that, by using the product (and by looking like her), others will become popular and successful.

Parents also have the responsibility of preparing their preteens for puberty and the physical transformation that will occur. For example, girls need to know that they will develop fat on their hips and other areas of their body, and that it is a normal part of development. They also need to be aware of growth spurts, and that hunger and increased appetite go along with them. As long as they eat a healthful diet and exercise, they do not need to worry about sudden weight gains during this time period. Furthermore, they should be aware that sometimes teens gain weight before they get taller.

The National Eating Disorders Association (NEDA) provides additional information for parents and others who work with children and teens. They stress the need for parents and others to be positive role models. Parents need to think about their own attitudes, beliefs, and behaviors and try to change those that are unhealthful. In addition, they must eliminate all preconceived perceptions of how they want their child to look or how much they want their child to weigh. Furthermore, parents should allow all types of food into their home, encourage their children to eat when they are hungry, and refrain from using food as a reward or punishment. Instead of concentrating on food, parents and other role models need to focus on building self-esteem and a sense of self-worth. It is important to stress the inner attributes of oneself and others, such as kindness, empathy, concern, knowledge, and loyalty. Parents ought to teach children how to think critically and question, rather than conform to peer pressure or be easily influenced by advertisements and mass media. Fathers, in particular, need to voice their desire and belief that role models should be similar for both women and men.

Children should learn about taking control of their health. For example, they should learn the importance of a varied, well-rounded diet and a healthy amount of exercise, but also about stress reduction and coping strategies, particularly when it concerns issues surrounding adolescence. They also need to be aware of the impact of dieting, which is seen as a precursor to the development of anorexia nervosa. They need to know the facts. NEDA attempts to take the glamour out of dieting by providing facts. The most important fact is that dieting almost never works, as 95% of dieters end up back at their initial weight or heavier.

Physicians can also help in terms of prevention and early detection. When they see patients for their yearly physicals, they should talk about the healthful approach to eating and exercising. They can also include a discussion regarding self-esteem and adolescence as the child approaches the teen years. Physicians should look at the weight and height each year, calculate the BMI and compare it to previous years. And they should ask questions about eating and exercise habits, satisfaction with body appearance, dieting, and excessive concern with weight. If there is the possibility of an eating disorder, the patient should return every week or two until the physician is certain whether or not to refer the patient for an evaluation.

FUTURE RESEARCH

Although there has been an explosion of research regarding anorexia over the past few decades, there is still much to be done. Overall, the cure rate is relatively low and the morbidity is high, especially in those who have had anorexia for more than three years or who are no longer young teens. Experts continue to debate the actual diagnosis of anorexia, questioning whether it is accurate, and whether more specific subgroups need to be defined so that better treatment recommendations can be made based on the subtype of anorexia. In addition, experts are attempting to identify programs that will decrease, rather than increase the risk of developing anorexia. Plus, they are evaluating screening tools which will help identify individuals at risk of developing anorexia, or those in the early stages of anorexia so that they can begin treatment as soon as possible. Furthermore, researchers are analyzing the various therapies, trying to find which will work best with specific groups of anorexics and which combinations of treatments and support services provide the best outcomes for the specific groups.

In addition to clinical studies, radiologic studies are also being evaluated with regard to anorexia. One important area of research is the use of neuroimaging techniques, or specific brain scans, to evaluate how anorexics process information both during their illness and after recovery. For example, they are being used to evaluate brain activity within specific regions of the brain. In addition, scans can help differentiate between short-term and chronic changes in brain receptor activity during illness and after recovery. In all of these studies, scans of those with anorexia are being compared to matched controls, or individuals without an eating disorder. Furthermore, researchers have begun to question the differences in brain structure and function between anorexics and those with other psychiatric illnesses, such as depressive disorders and obsessive-compulsive disorder. The researchers hope to find common abnormalities with the other disorders so they can then target drug treatments (Frank et al. 2004).

Another important area of research is the possibility that anorexia, or the risk of developing anorexia, could be inherited. Scientists are looking at genetic material to try to identify similar patterns in individuals with anorexia. Eventually, they hope to determine the underlying cause of the illness so they can find an appropriate, successful treatment for it (APA Steering Committee on Practice Guidelines 2006).

A final important area of research with regard to anorexia is that of medications. Obviously, the goal is to find medications which can either increase weight gain or treat several symptoms of anorexia. While several medications have already been tested on patients with anorexia, they have not been very successful. Several new drugs which were developed are currently in clinical trials. Many of the drugs being tested were recruited because of specific findings from neuroimaging studies. Such studies have demonstrated how various neurotransmitters and receptors function within the brain of an anorexic. The list of drugs currently or soon to be in clinical trials is long and complex. It includes neuropeptide antagonists, orexin receptor antagonists, corticotropin-releasing factor receptor 2 antagonists, histamine 3 antagonists, melanocortin 4 receptor antagonists, beta 3-adrenoceptor agonists, 5-hydroxytryptamine-2A antagonists, and growth hormone agonists. These medications are being evaluated to determine their success on a variety of symptoms of anorexia. Some of the results they are looking for include decreased delusional thoughts surrounding eating, stimulation of the hunger response, quicker time for food to leave the stomach, increased metabolic rate, changes in the regulation of food intake, and stimulation and improvement in the energy balance (Steffen et al. 2006).

A little over a century ago, the term *anorexia nervosa* was just being defined. Since that period, we have learned a great deal about those who have this specific eating disorder. Yet there is still much more to discover. For example, while treatments have been successful with specific groups of anorexics, they are still inadequate as a whole. In addition, medications have not yet been shown to alleviate major symptoms of anorexia. Furthermore, we still have not determined the best methods to keep teens from developing anorexia. These are all important areas of current and future research in the field of eating disorders.

Timeline of Anorexia Nervosa

1st–5th centuries	Cases of men and women practicing self-starvation mainly for religious or medical reasons
383 AD	Follower of St. Jerome starves herself to death
6th–11th centuries	Scattered cases of self-starvation during Dark Ages, possibly due to fewer fasters or lack of adequate documentation
13th century	Cases of (mostly) women starving themselves for religious and ascetic reasons, termed "Holy Anorexics"
1347	Birth of Catherine of Siena, a holy anorexic who became a Saint, which is typical of that epoch
15th–16th centuries	Cases of self-starvation attributed to demonic possession or bewitchment
1689	Dr. Richard Morton gives first medical description of what may be modern-day anorexia nervosa when he writes about "nervous consumption" caused by sadness and anxious cares in *Phthisiologia: A Treatise of Consumption*

17th–19th centuries	Era of "miraculous maidens," where no known cause, such as religion or possession, can be attributed to self-starvation in (mainly) women
1764	Robert Whytt documents biological changes that occur within the body with severe fasting and starvation
Early 19th century	Era of Scientific Revolution, when physicians and others begin to question authenticity of miraculous maidens and attempt to prove their fraudulence, such as occurred with Anne Moore of Tutbury and Sarah Jacobs, the "Welsh Fasting Girl"
1859–1860	Physicians William Stout Chipley, Pierre Briquet, and Louis-Victor Marcé independently write about women who starve themselves and document differences between various groups of women, such as those who lack any other medical illness yet refuse to eat
1868	Sir William Gull during a speech at the annual meeting of the British Medical Association in England discusses several cases of healthy young women starving themselves
1873	Charles Lasègue publishes his paper, "On Hysterical Anorexia," where he discusses, in detail, psychological aspects of anorexia, such as family struggles
1873	Sir William Gull coins and becomes the first physician to use the term "anorexia nervosa," and to describe the illness as a unique medical condition
1890s	Famous graphic artist, Dana Gibson, creates the Gibson Girl that replaces drawings of full-figure women with a slimmer prototype
1900s	Parisian fashion designs, emphasizing slimness and small busts, make their way into the fashion industry
1914	Morris Simmonds categorizes most women who starve themselves as having Simmonds' disease, an atrophy of the anterior pituitary gland. Major treatments for self-starvation become hormonal therapy, such as thyroid and growth hormone
1918	Lulu Hunt Peters writes the first bestselling book about weight loss and dieting
1920s	Standard dress sizes are introduced

1930s	Simmonds' disease is discounted as sole cause of self-starvation
1940s	Freud's "oral impregnation theory" of self-starvation becomes popular
1944	The first edition of *Seventeen* magazine is published. The magazine, geared toward teens, emphasizes slimness, dieting, and beauty
1950s	Diet foods are widely advertised in the media
1960s–1980s	Well-known experts, such as Hilde Bruch, Mara Selvini-Palazzoli, and Gerald Russell, theorize that anorexia nervosa is mainly due to dysfunctional family dynamics
1966	English supermodel Lesley Hornby, nicknamed Twiggy, arrives in the United States. At 5'7" and 90 pounds, she radically alters the fashion industry and becomes a role model for extreme thinness
1970s	Anorexia Nervosa becomes focus of many newspaper and magazine articles, TV shows, movies, and books, including Hilde Bruch's book, *The Golden Cage: The Enigma of Anorexia Nervosa*
1976	The establishment of the National Association of Anorexia Nervosa and Associated Disorders
1980s	Development of a team model approach for anorexia nervosa which includes several specialists working with the anorexic, such as nutritionists, psychologists, family therapists, and nurses
1980	Eating disorders are officially recognized as a mental illness in the psychiatric reference book, the *Diagnostic Statistics Manual, Third Revision*
1981	First issue of the *International Journal of Eating Disorders* is published
1981	TV movie, based on the book, *The Best Little Girl in the World*, increases awareness and comprehension of anorexia nervosa in the United States
February 4, 1983	Karen Carpenter, a beloved and renowned singer, dies from heart failure as a result of anorexia nervosa

1985	Renfrew Center, the first residential treatment facility serving only those with eating disorders opens in Philadelphia, Pennsylvania
1993	The Academy for Eating Disorders forms after a meeting with 33 clinicians and researchers specializing in eating disorders The American Psychiatric Association publishes its first set of practice guidelines for the treatment of anorexia nervosa
August 21, 1994	Gymnast Christy Henrich dies from organ failure as a result of anorexia nervosa
Late 1990s	The emergence of a pro-eating disorder culture ("pro-ana") on the Internet with forums, clubs, and chat groups to encourage and support others who want to maintain an eating disorder
1999	Average female television actress is 3″ taller and 40 pounds lighter than the average American woman
2001	The National Eating Disorders Association is formed Development of "Maudsley Method," a popular new approach to treating adolescents with anorexia nervosa
2002	International team of researchers publish a paper identifying a region on chromosome 1 as being potentially related to the development of anorexia nervosa

2006	Fashion model Ana Carolina Reston dies from complications secondary to anorexia nervosa and bulimia nervosa
	     Fashion model Luisel Ramos dies of heart failure secondary to malnutrition as a result of anorexia nervosa, and her sister, Eliana, also a model, dies less than a year later from complications of anorexia nervosa
	     Fashion designers in Spain decide to set a minimum BMI of 18 for all models participating in Madrid Fashion Week, while Italian Fashion designers require a minimum BMI of 18.5, a certificate of health from a physician, and a minimum age of 16 to walk down their runway.
	     Popular antidepressant, Prozac, is found not to be useful in treating anorexia nervosa

2007	Over 500 pro-anorexia Web sites exist on the Internet 11.7 million cosmetic surgical and nonsurgical procedures are done in the United States and over $7 billion is spent on cosmetics alone

Online Information and Support for Anorexia Nervosa

National Institute of Mental Health (NIMH), National Institutes of Health (NIH), Health and Human Services (HHS)

Phone: (866) 615-NIMH (6464)

Internet Address: http://www.nimh.nih.gov

The largest scientific organization in the world which provides scientific, objective information on understanding, treating, and preventing mental illnesses, including anorexia nervosa.

National Mental Health Information Center, Substance Abuse and Mental Health Services Administration (SAMHSA), HHS

Phone: (800) 789-2647

Internet Address: http://www.mentalhealth.org

Provides quality information and resources on anorexia nervosa.

National Association of Anorexia Nervosa and Associated Disorders

Phone: (847) 831-3438

Internet Address: http://www.anad.org

Involved in many activities related to anorexia nervosa, including providing a 24-hour hotline, educating the public and professionals, and helping to locate therapists and support groups. They are also heavily involved in consumer advocacy and legislation in an attempt to prevent anorexia nervosa and adequately treat those who have it.

National Eating Disorders Association

Phone: (800) 931-2237

Internet Address: http://www.nationaleatingdisorders.org

Provides education, resources, and support to individuals, family members, friends, and professionals. Provides toolkits filled with helpful information for parents and educators.

Something Fishy Web site on Eating Disorders

Phone: (866) 690-7239

Internet Address: http://www.something-fishy.org/

Raises awareness and provides support to those with eating disorders and their families. Helps locate a provider.

Eating Disorders Awareness and Prevention, Inc.

Phone: (800) 931-2237 or (206) 382-3587

Internet Address: http://www.edap.org

Academy for Eating Disorders

Phone: (847) 498-4274

Internet Address: http://www.aedweb.org

Provides professional training and education, encourages new developments in research, prevention, and clinical treatment. Is a source for the most current information regarding eating disorders.

Eating Disorder Referral and Information Center

Phone: (858) 792-7463

Internet Address: http://www.edreferral.com

Provides information and resources for the treatment of eating disorders. Also helps with locating professionals in the field of eating disorders.

Glossary

Abstinence—to refrain from various pleasures such as food, alcohol, and sexual relations

Acrocyanosis—a blueness of the fingers and toes, which is a sign of poor circulation or decreased blood flow to these areas of the body

Amenorrhea—the lack of three menstrual cycles, or periods, in a row in females

Anemia—a lower than normal amount of hemoglobin in the body to make red blood cells, leading to problems such as tiredness, weakness, shortness of breath, and pallor

Anorexia—"loss of appetite"

Antipsychotic—a medication used to treat certain mental illnesses, such as schizophrenia, to inhibit abnormal thoughts or fixed beliefs

Apepsia—a term used frequently in the 1800s to describe women who reportedly had weak digestive systems, which led to a host of medical complaints and symptoms

Arrhythmia—abnormal conduction of the heart beat or electrical impulse within the heart, where the conduction may not follow the regular pathway or may have abnormal timing

Ascetism—the pursuit of perfection of the spiritual life in the Christian tradition

Asexuality—a lack of sexual desire

Atrophy (of brain)—wasting or shrinkage of areas of the brain

Binge—eating large, excessive amounts of food in a small period of time

Blood pressure—the force of blood against the inner walls of the blood vessels, or the pressure required to push blood through the body during the different phases of heart contraction, which can vary during different states of health

Body mass index (BMI)—a calculation of weight for height (weight in kg/(height in meters)^2), based on age and sex, which provides information on whether someone is overweight, underweight, or normal weight

Bone marrow—the tissue in the middle of bones which makes red blood cells, white blood cells, and platelets

Bradycardia—a slow heart rate of less than 60 beats per minute

Bulimia nervosa—an eating disorder mainly affecting young women, where they regularly and repeatedly binge and then purge to avoid weight gain

Calcium—a vital element in the body, which is a major component of bones and teeth, and is necessary for functions such as normal nerve conduction, heart conduction, and muscle contraction

Carbohydrates—compounds that we eat, such as pasta, bread, and rice, which provide energy for our bodies

Cardiomyopathy—a disease of the heart muscle which leads to decreased ability of the heart to contract and function normally

Chlorosis—a term used in the 20th century to describe someone with a green pallor due to iron deficiency anemia; typically attacks females after onset of puberty

Coma—a state of unconsciousness, where the person is completely unresponsive and unarousable

Co-morbid—having more than one diagnosis, or problem, at the same time

Consumption—a term used commonly in the 1900s to describe someone who had a disease which led to wasting of the body, particularly when referring to tuberculosis

Core body temperature—the normal body temperature in a healthy, resting individual, which is 37 degrees Celsius or 98.6 degrees Fahrenheit

Cortisol—a steroid hormone produced by the adrenal cortex near the kidneys which regulates carbohydrate metabolism and the body's normal response to internal and external stresses

Crohn's disease—a chronic, sometimes debilitating inflammatory condition involving the gastrointestinal tract, most commonly the small and large intestines; it leads to swelling and sores or ulcers within the intestines which can cause life-threatening complications

Cyproheptadine—a medication used to treat allergies, such as hay fever, which is also used experimentally to stimulate the appetite

Cysapride—a medication which improves gastric motility, or the movement of food through the stomach; no longer available in the United States

Delusion—a false, fixed belief, such as believing that you are receiving messages through the television

Diabetes mellitus—a condition which leads to excessive amounts of sugar, or glucose, in the blood and urine because of the inability to store it in the body; without treatment it can lead to permanent damage and complications in the body, or even death

Distorted body image—false image of one's body, such as the belief that one is obese when they are in fact very underweight

Diuretic—a medication used to rid the body of excess urine

DSM—diagnostic statistical manual, the authoritative book for mental health professionals that provides lists and explanations of mental disorders and requirements necessary to make the diagnosis; used in the United States and other parts of the world

Dyspepsia—pain or discomfort in the lower chest, indicative of esophageal pain, which can be accompanied by nausea and vomiting

Electrolyte shift—movement of electrolytes from inside a cell to outside a cell, or vice versa, to try to maintain normal levels within the body

Electrolytes—the amount, or concentration, of essential ions in the blood and tissues needed to maintain fluid balance and functions within the body; sodium, potassium, chloride, and calcium are examples of electrolytes

Endocrine system—the system of endocrine glands within the body which release hormones to regulate activities, such as blood pressure, body temperature, and growth

Endorphin—a group of hormones in the brain that decrease pain sensation and affect emotions

Endoscopy—a procedure performed by a gastroenterologist, where a special scope is inserted into the intestines or esophagus to view it and obtain tissue samples

Enema—a fluid injected into the rectum to cause a bowel movement

ESR (erythrocyte sedimentation rate)—a blood test which provides general information as to whether there may be an inflammatory condition within the body

Estrogen/estradiol—major female sex hormones which contribute to the development and maintenance of reproductive capabilities

Eucharist—Holy Communion, a way to receive Jesus' invisible presence in the form of bread and wine

Fluoxetine—an antidepressant in the SSRI class (see SSRI)

Follicular stimulating hormone (FSH)—a hormone released by the anterior pituitary gland in the brain which is partially responsible for initiation and maintenance of pregnancy

Genetic—inherited, in genetic material

Ghrelin—a hormone produced in the stomach and pancreas which stimulates appetite and increases food intake; it is also produced in the hypothalamus within the brain and causes the release of growth hormone

Green sickness—chlorosis; a term used in the 20th century to describe someone with a green pallor due to iron deficiency anemia; typically attacks females after onset of puberty

Growth hormone—a hormone produced in the anterior pituitary gland that causes growth of the long bones, such as the arms and legs

Hallucination—a false belief that something is present, through seeing, hearing, smelling, tasting, or feeling something that doesn't exist

Heart failure—the inability of the heart to function normally

Heredity—the passage of genes from parents to children

Holy anorexic—the term coined by historian, Rudolph Bell, to describe women who practiced self-starvation and devoted their lives to the Church during the Middle Ages

Hormone—a substance made in the body which travels through the bloodstream to other areas to produce an effect, such as a feeling of hunger or an increase in heart rate

Human genome—the entire map of DNA, consisting of 23 pairs of chromosomes, which makes us human beings

Hyperalimentation—the process of providing nutrients and calories through an intravenous line in those who refuse or are unable to take it through other methods, such as the mouth or stomach

Hyponatremia—low sodium level in the blood, which can cause dehydration, brain swelling, seizures, coma, and other problems

Hypothalamus—an area in the brain that produces and releases hormones to regulate temperature, appetite, thirst, sexual function, and sleep, in addition to other functions

Hypothermia—when the body's temperature falls below that necessary for normal functioning; this can occur after the body is exposed to a cold environment for a prolonged period, or when the body tries to conserve energy

Hysteria—acting with uncontrollable emotions, overly excited; a term often used to describe women who had physical complaints in the latter half of the 20th century

ICD—international statistical classification of diseases and related health problems, which is published by the World Health Organization; an authoritative reference book for clinicians to define and diagnose mental conditions; used by many professionals in Europe and other parts of the world

Ideal body weight (IBW)—the recommended body weight for males and females of different heights, which is indicative of the appropriate amount of body fat

Immune function—the ability of our body to fight off infections

Insulin—a hormone produced in the pancreas which regulates glucose and other nutrients within our body; it is absent in insulin-dependent diabetes mellitus, requiring those with this illness to give themselves insulin through a needle several times a day

Insulin-dependent diabetes—see diabetes mellitus

Ketoacidosis—a condition which occurs mainly in insulin-dependent diabetics, but can occur in other conditions such as dehydration, where ketone bodies build up in the bloodstream and cause acidosis, a dangerous drop in the pH of the blood

Laxative—a medicine that helps loosen and rid the body of stool; used for constipation

Leptin—a hormone produced in adipose (fat) tissue which causes us to feel full

Libido—sex drive

Lupus—an autoimmune disease, where the body attacks itself, causing chronic inflammation in many parts of the body, leading to pain and damage, especially in the kidneys, joints, blood and skin

Luteinizing hormone (LH)—a hormone produced and secreted by the anterior pituitary gland which causes women to ovulate and helps maintain a pregnancy; in males it leads to the production of testosterone

Magnetic resonance spectroscopy—a study where special imaging techniques are used to determine the concentration of certain chemicals within the brain; used to evaluate central nervous system disorders

Mallory-Weiss tear—a tear in the esophagus usually due to forceful vomiting or coughing; can lead to significant bleeding and blood loss

Malnutrition—the lack of a proper or balanced diet

Melanocortin—a hormone which has many roles, including that of appetite and satiety

Menarche—the date of the first menstrual period in females

Menses—flow of blood from the uterus; periods

Metabolic rate—the amount of energy the body uses in a fixed time period

Metabolism—the sum of all the physical and chemical changes that occur in a body and allow it to grow and function

Miraculous maiden—a term coined to describe females who fasted around the 1500s for no obvious reason, such as without a religious or medical explanation

Mysticism—a religious belief and desire to unify with the divine, or to try to become one with some divine or universal principle

Nasogastric feeding—providing liquid nutrition through a tube which is inserted through the nose into the stomach

Nervosa—"nervous"

Neuroimaging—the use of a variety of techniques to obtain direct or indirect images of the brain's structure, function, and pharmacology

Neurotransmitter—chemicals released from one neuron in the brain which send a signal or message to other neurons

Obsessive-compulsive disorder—an anxiety disorder which includes unwanted, persistent thoughts and repetitive behaviors; compulsions or rituals are often used to relieve the anxious thoughts

Olanzapine—an atypical antipsychotic medication which also causes weight gain; used in experimental studies to try to stimulate the appetite

Organic brain syndrome—a term used for both short-term and long-term disorders that cause problems with mental function; this can cause confusion, problems with memory, difficulty concentrating and performing various mental tasks

Orthostatic hypotension—a sudden drop in blood pressure which occurs with standing after being in a sitting or lying position; can cause dizziness or feeling of faintness

Osteopenia—a decrease in bone mass or bone density which, if untreated, can lead to osteoporosis

Osteoporosis—a disease where there is significant loss of bone mass, leading to very brittle and porous bones and predisposing to fractures and chronic bone pain

Parotid gland—a salivary gland which secretes saliva into the mouth; it can become swollen with repeated episodes of purging

Peripheral neuropathy—damage to the nerves that send messages to and from the spinal cord

Phosphate—an ion needed for maintenance of healthy bones and for normal functioning of cells; high levels can lead to organ damage and other effects due to its direct relationship to calcium

Phrenology—a popular theory in the 1800s that the shape of the skull represents specific mental abilities and personality characteristics

Pituitary gland—a gland in the base of the brain which produces and secretes many hormones, including growth hormone, LH, FSH, ACTH, TSH, and others which are responsible for functions such as puberty, reproductive capability, growth, sleep, and appetite

Platelets—cells made by the bone marrow which help with clotting of blood

Positron emission tomography—a nuclear medicine imaging technique that evaluates blood flow and metabolic activity in a specified organ, particularly helpful in evaluating metabolic activity within the brain

Potassium—an electrolyte which plays an important role in muscular contraction, including those of the heart and gastrointestinal system; low potassium levels can cause problems such as muscle cramps, stomach pain, and abnormal contraction of the heart; both high and low levels can lead to death

Psychiatrist—a medical doctor who provides therapy and prescribes medication for people with mental illnesses and other emotional issues

Psychoanalysis—a type of therapeutic intervention where a psychiatrist tries to help uncover unconscious thoughts, feelings, and conflicts which contribute to current issues; the person is said to be undergoing psychotherapy

Psychologist—a PhD or PsyD who has received several years of training and clinical experience beyond undergraduate school and provides therapy for individuals with mental and emotional problems

Psychosis—one aspect of several mental disorders which includes hallucinations and delusions, where one has an altered sense of reality

Pubertal growth spurt—the period during adolescence where there is rapid height growth

Puberty—adolescence; the time during which the body changes to become one of reproductive capability and to look like that of an adult

Purge—the act of making oneself throw up food contents

Receptor—a protein on the surface of a cell where a molecule, such as a hormone or neurotransmitter, binds to cause a predictable response by that cell, such as a feeling of hunger or the production of sperm

Reformation—changes made by the Catholic Church, including spiritual, religious, and political elements, beginning around the mid 16th century

Renfrew Center—The country's first residential treatment center for eating disorders, which opened in 1985 in Philadelphia

Revelation—the act of communication with God, disclosure of information to humans by God

Sacraments—church rituals, such as Holy Communion

Satiety—feeling full, lack of hunger

Seizure—an abnormal firing of neurons from the brain which can cause a loss of consciousness and uncontrollable spasms, or the feeling of different sensations and uncontrollable movements of specific body parts

Selective serotonin reuptake inhibitor (SSRI)—a class of medications which increases the amount of serotonin in the brain which may decrease feelings of depression and anxiety, in addition to other undesired emotions

Self-castigation—punishing oneself severely, mentally or physically, to prove devotion to God or to strive to become religiously pure

Serotonin—a neurotransmitter which is involved in many phenomena originating in the brain, including mood, appetite, sleep, memory and learning, and sexual desire

Sex steroids—the main steroids, or hormones, that produce the direct effects on our bodies are estrogen, for women, and testosterone, for men; although other steroids such as LH and FSH regulate estrogen and testosterone

Simmonds' disease—a dysfunction of the anterior part of the pituitary gland which leads to atrophy of many organs, including the heart, thyroid, and adrenal glands; those affected lose weight and become malnourished

Sitomania—an abnormal craving for food

Sitophobia—a "morbid" aversion to food; a term commonly used in the late 1800s to describe (mainly) females who did not eat for a variety of reasons

Social worker—someone who has received a master's degree in social work (MSW) and has learned how to counsel patients to help them improve their lives

Sodium—an element which maintains water and electrolyte balance in the body; both too much and too little sodium, such as can occur with dehydration or water overload, can lead to problems including seizures, brain swelling, heart arrhythmias, and death

Testosterone—the main sex hormone in males responsible for most of the changes which occur in males during puberty

Thin ideal—an unrealistic goal of trying to look like ultra-thin women in the media

Thyroid hormone—produced by the thyroid and has several critical functions, including regulation of the basal metabolic rate, body temperature, and metabolism of protein, fat, and carbohydrates

Tricyclic antidepressant—a medication used to treat depression which is not used as much now as it was before the advent of SSRIs

Tuberculosis—a serious infectious disease which usually affects the lungs but can occur anywhere in the body; it can lay dormant in the body for years and then resurface and, without long-term appropriate antibiotics, can lead to death; it was very common before the age of antibiotics and still is in underdeveloped communities

Ventricles (in brain)—the areas of the brain where cerebrospinal fluid flows

Westernization—the influence and practice of ideas, cultures, and customs from the United States, Great Britain, and other wealthy countries

White blood cells—cells which are produced mainly in the bone marrow and are responsible for fighting off infections

Bibliography

American Academy of Pediatrics Committee on Adolescence. "Identifying and Treating Eating Disorders: Committee on Adolescence Policy Statement." *Pediatrics* 111, no. 1 (2003): 204–211.

American Psychiatric Association. *Diagnostic and Statistical Manual of Mental Disorders*, Fourth Edition, Text Revision. Washington, DC: American Psychiatric Association Press, 2000.

American Psychiatric Association. "Practice Guidelines for the Treatment of Patients with Eating Disorders, Third Edition." In American Psychiatric Association Practice Guidelines for the Treatment of Psychiatric Disorders: Compendium 2006, 1097–1222. Arlington, VA: American Psychiatric Publishing, Inc., 2006.

Anorexia Nervosa and Associated Eating Disorders. Facts about Eating Disorders. http://www.anad.org (accessed April 2008).

Anorexia Nervosa and Related Eating Disorders. Diabetes and Eating Disorders. http://www.anred.com/diab.html (accessed April 2008).

———. Males with Eating Disorders. http://www.anred.com/males.html (accessed July 25, 2008).

———. Statistics: How Many People Have Eating Disorders? http://www.anred.com/stats.html (accessed April 2008).

Anorexia Nervosa and Related Eating Disorders. Eating Disorders Warning Signs. http://www.anred.com/warn.html (accessed April 2008).

The Anorexic Queen. April 16, 2008. http://community.livejournal.com/anorexicqueen (accessed April 16, 2008).

APA Steering Committee on Practice Guidelines. Treatment of Patients with Eating Disorders. American Psychiatric Association Practice Guidelines, Arlington, VA: APA, 2006.

Bardone-Cone, A.M., and K.M. Cass. "What Does Viewing a Pro-Anorexia Website Do? An Experimental Examination of Website Exposure and Moderating Effects." *International Journal of Eating Disorders* 40, no. 6 (2007): 537–548.

Becker, A., R. Burwell, D. Herzog, and P. Hamburg. "Eating Behaviors and Attitudes Following Prolonged Exposure to Television among Ethnic Fijian Adolescent Girls." *British Journal of Psychiatry* 180 (2002): 509–514.

Bell, Rudolph. *Holy Anorexia.* Chicago: University of Chicago Press, 1985.

Bemporad, J. "Self-Starvation through the Ages: Reflections on the Pre-History of Anorexia Nervosa." *International Journal of Eating Disorders* 19, no. 3 (1996): 217–237.

Berkman, N., et al. Management of Eating Disorders. Evidence Report/Technology Assessment No. 135. AHRQ Publication No. 06-E010, University of North Carolina Evidence-Based Practice Center, University of North Carolina, Rockville, MD: Agency for Healthcare Research and Quality, 2006.

Berkman, N., K. Lohr, and C. Bulik. "Outcomes of Eating Disorders: A Systematic Review of the Literature." *International Journal of Eating Disorders* 40, no. 4 (2007): 293–309.

Bhanji, S., and B.B. Newton. "Richard Morton's Account of Nervous Consumption." *International Journal of Eating Disorders* 4 (1985): 589–595.

Blum, Sam. "Children Who Starve Themselves." *The New York Times*, November 10, 1974.

Braun, Devra. "Which Males Develop Eating Disorders?" *Medscape Psychiatry & Mental Health eJournal* 2, no. 2 (1997).

Bruch, Hilde. *Conversations with Anorexics.* Edited by Danita Czyzewski and Melanie Suhr. New York: Basic Books, Inc., 1988.

Bruch, Hilde. *Eating Disorders: Obesity, Anorexia Nervosa, and the Person Within.* New York: Basic Books, Inc., 1973.

———. *The Golden Cage: The Enigma of Anorexia Nervosa.* Cambridge: Harvard University Press, 1978.

Brumberg, Joan Jacobs. *Fasting Girls: The History of Anorexia.* New York: Vintage Books, 2000.

———. *The Body Project: An Intimate History of American Girls.* New York: Vintage Books, 1997.

Bulik, C.M., N.D. Berkman, K. Brownley, J.A. Sedway, and K.N. Lohr. "Anorexia Nervosa Treatment: A Systematic Review of Randomized Controlled Trials." *International Journal of Eating Disorders* 40, no. 4 (2007): 310–320.

Caringonline. Celebrities with Eating Disorders. http://caringonline.com/eatdis/people. htm (accessed April 18, 2008).

Carter, Jacqueline, Anne Stewart, Valerie Dunn, and Christopher Fairburn. "Primary Prevention of Eating Disorders: Might It Do More Harm Than Good?" *International Journal of Eating Disorders* 2, no. 22 (1998): 167–172.

Castro-Fornieles, J., et al. "Predictors of Weight Maintenance after Hospital Discharge in Adolescents with Anorexia Nervosa." *International Journal of Eating Disorders* 39 (2006): 212–216.

Catholic Information Network. Catherine of Siena, 1347–1380. http://www.cin.org/ saints/cathsiena.html (accessed February 2008).

Chafe, William. *The Paradox of Change: American Women in the 20th Century.* New York: Oxford University Press, 1992.

Chao, Y., et al. "Ethnic Differences in Weight Control Practices among U.S. Adolescents from 1995 to 2005" *International Journal of Eating Disorders* 48 (2008): 124–133.

Cohn, Leigh. Fat Is Not Just a Feminine Issue Anymore. 2000. http://ww.gurze.com/ client/client_pages/abouteating_males.cfm (accessed April 11, 2008).

Colahan, Mireille, and Paul Robinson. "Multi-Family Groups in the Treatment of Young Adults with Eating Disorders." *Journal of Family Therapy* 24, no. 1 (February 2002): 17.

Commission on Adolescent Eating Disorders. "Treating and Preventing Adolescent Mental Health Disorders." In *Treating and Preventing Adolescent Mental Health Disorders*, edited by Dwight Evans, et al., 255–329. Oxford: Oxford University Press, 2007.

Couturier, J., and J. Lock. "What Is Recovery in Adolescent Anorexia Nervosa?" *International Journal of Eating Disorders* 39, no. 7 (2006a): 550–555.

Couturier, J., and J. Lock. "Denial and Minimization in Adolescents with Anorexia Nervosa." *International Journal of Eating Disorders* 39 (2006b): 454–461.

Crisp, Arthur. "In Defense of the Concept of Phobically Driven Avoidance of Adult Body Weight/Shape/Function as the Final Common Pathway to Anorexia Nervosa." *European Eating Disorders Review* 14 (2006): 189–202.

Cunningham, Patricia A. *Reforming Women's Fashion, 1850–1920: Politics, Health and Art.* Kent: Kent State University Press, 2003.

Dare, Christopher, Eleni Chania, Ivan Eisler, Matthew Hodes, Elizabeth Dodge, and Christopher Dare. "The Eating Disorder Inventory as an Instrument to Explore change in Adolescents in Family Therapy for Anorexia Nervosa." *European Eating Disorders Review* 8, no. 5 (2000): 369–383.

Evans, D., et al. *Treating and Preventing Adolescent Mental Health Disorders.* Oxford: Oxford University Press, 2007.

Farah, Mounir, and Andrea Berens Karls. World History: The Human Experience. New York: McGraw-Hill Companies, Inc., 2001.

Fichter, M., N. Quadflieg, and S. Hedlund. "Twelve-Year Course and Outcome Predictors of Anorexia Nervosa." *International Journal of Eating Disorders* 39 (2006): 87–100.

Field, Alison, Lilian Cheung, Anne Wolf, David Herzog, Steven Gortmaker, and Graham Colditz. "Exposure to the Mass Media and Weight Concerns among Girls." *Pediatrics* 103, no. 3 (1999): e36.

Fisher, Martin. "Treatment of Eating Disorders in Children, Adolescents, and Young Adults." *Pediatrics in Review* 27 (2006): 5–16.

Frank, G., U. Bailer, S. Henry, A. Wagner, and W. Kaye. "Neuroimaging Studies in Eating Disorders." *CNS Spectrums* 9, no. 7 (2004): 539–548.

Franko, D., A. Becker, J. Thomas, and D. Herzog. "Cross-Ethnic Differences in Eating Disorder Symptoms and Related Distress." *International Journal of Eating Disorders* 34, no. 4 (2007): 156–164.

Frisch, M., D. Herzog, and D. Franko. "Residential Treatment for Eating Disorders." *International Journal of Eating Disorders* 39, no. 5 (2006): 434–442.

Gold, Tracy, and Julie McCarron. *Room to Grow: An Appetite for Life.* Beverly Hills: New Millennium Press, 2003.

Good, Erica. "The Male Battle with Anorexia." *The New York Times*, July 25, 2008.

Gordon, Richard. *Eating Disorders: Anatomy of a Social Epidemic.* Malden, MA: Blackwell Publishers Ltd., 2000.

Gottlieb, Lori. *Stick Figure.* New York: Simon & Schuster, 2000.

Gowers, S.G., et al. "Treatment Aims and Philosophy in the Treatment of Adolescent Anorexia Nervosa in Europe." *European Eating Disorders Review* 10 (2002): 271–280.

Gura, Trish. *Lying in Weight: The Hidden Epidemic of Eating Disorders in Adult Women.* New York: HarperCollins Publishers, 2007.

Habermas, T. "On the Uses of History in Psychiatry: Diagnostic Implications for Anorexia Nervosa." *International Journl of Eating Disorders* 38 (2005): 167–182.

Hargreaves, D., and M. Tiggemann. "Body Image Is for Girls: A Qualitative Study of Boys' Body Image." *Journal of Health Psychology* 11, no. 4 (2006): 567–576.

Hargrove, JL. "History of the Calorie in Nutrition." *Journal of Nutrition* 136, no. 12 (December 2006): 2957–2961.

Harrison, K. "Television Viewers' Ideal Body Proportions: The Case of the Curvaceously Thin Woman." *Sex Roles* 48, no. 5/6 (2003): 255.

Harrison, K. "Does Interpersonal Attraction to Thin Media Personalities Promote Eating Disorders?" *Journal of Broadcasting and Electronic Media* 41, no. 4 (1997): 478.

Harrison, K., and J. Cantor. "The Relationship between Media Consumption and Eating Disorders." *Journal of Communication* 47, no. 1 (1997): 40.

Haug, Joanne. Dressing up: Women's Fashions 1855–1860. http://www.victoriana.com/1850sfashion/victorianfashionhistoroy1850.htm (accessed March 2008).

Hesse-Biber, Sharlene. *Am I Thin Enough Yet? The Cult of Thinness and the Commercialization of Identity.* New York: Oxford University Press, 1997.

Hill, Michael. Male Eating Disorders on the Rise. May 11, 2004. http://www.gurze.com/client/client_pages/aparticle.cfm (accessed April 8, 2008).

History of Beauty. http://inventors.about.com/library/inventors/blbeauty.com (accessed April 4, 2008).

Kaibara, A., et al. "Leptin Produces Anorexia and Weight Loss without Inducing an Acute Phase Response or Protein Wasting." *American Journal of Physiology* 274, no. 6 (1998): R1518–R1525.

Kaye, W. "Neurobiology of Anorexia and Bulimia Nervosa." *Physiology & Behavior* 94, no. 1 (2008): 121–135.

Kaye, W.H., et al. "Serotonin Alterations in Anorexia and Bulimia Nervosa: New Insights from Imaging Studies." *Physiology & Behavior* 85, no. 1 (2005): 73–81.

Keel, P., and K. Klump. "Are Eating Disorders Culture-Bound Syndromes? Implications for Conceptualizing their Etiology." *Psychological Bulletin* 129, no. 5 (2003): 747–769.

Landau, Elaine. *Why Are They Starving Themselves?* New York: Julian Messner, a Division of Simon Schuster, Inc., 1983.

Lawrence, C., and M. Thelen. "Body Image, Dieting and Self-Concept: Their Relation in African-American and Caucasian Children." *Journal of Clinical Child Psychology* 24 (1995): 41–48.

Laycock, Thomas. *A Treatise on the Nervous Diseases of Women; Comprising an Inquiry into the Nature, Causes and Treatment of Spinal and Hysterical Disorders.* London: Longmans, 1840.

Le Grange, Daniel, and James Lock. "Family-Based Treatment of Adolescent Anorexia Nervosa: The Maudsley Approach." NEDIC. http://www.nedic.ca (accessed June 2008).

Levenkron, Steven. *Anatomy of Anorexia.* New York: WW Norton and Company, Inc., 2000.

———. *The Best Little Girl in the World.* New York: Warner Brothers, Inc., 1978.

Levey, Robert. "Anorexia Nervosa." WebMD. http://www.emedicine.com/med/topic144.htm (accessed April 25, 2008).

Linblad, F., L. Lindberg, and A. Hjern. "Anorexia Nervosa in Young Men: A Cohort Study." *International Journal of Eating Disorders* 39, no. 8 (2006): 662–666.

Lindberg, L., and A. Hjern. "Risk Factors for Anorexia Nervosa: A National Cohort Study." *International Journal of Eating Disorders* 34, no. 4 (2003): 397–408.

Linton, Elizabeth Lynn. "Jane Stretton and the Cunning Woman." In *Witch Stories,* by Elizabeth Lynn Linton, 298–301. London: Chatto and Windus, 1883.

Lucas, Alexander. *Demystifying Anorexia Nervosa: An Optimistic Guide to Understanding and Healing.* Oxford: Oxford University Press, 2004.

MacKenzie, John. "The Victorian Vision: Inventing New Britain." *History Today* 51 (April 2001).

Malson, Carol. *The Thin Woman: Feminism, Post-Structuralism, and the Social Psychology of Anorexia Nerovsa.* New York: Routledge, 1998.

Marcus, Cherie. The Thinning of Women. November 30, 2000. http://iml.jou.ufl.edu/projects/Fall2000/Marcus/disorders2.htm (accessed April 11, 2008).

Martinez-Gonzalez, M., P. Gual, F. Lahortiga, Y. Alonso, J. Irala-Estevez, and S. Servera. "Mass Media Influences, and the Onset of Eating Disorders in a Prospective Population-Based Cohort." *Pediatrics* 111, no. 2 (2003): 315–320.

McGregor-Wood, Simon, and Karen Mooney. "Did Model Die from Pressure to Be Thin?" *ABC News*, November 19, 2007.

McIntosh, V., J. Jordan, S. Luty, F., McKenzie, J. Carter, C. Bulik, and P. Joyce. "Specialist Supportive Clinical Management for Anorexia Nervosa." *International Journal of Eating Disorders* 39, no. 8 (2006): 625–633.

Media Awareness Network. Beauty and Body Image in the Media. http://www.media-awareness.ca/english/issues/stereotyping/women_and_girls/women_beauty.cfm (accessed April 2008).

Miljic, D., et al. "Ghrelin has Partial or no Effect on Appetite, Growth Hormone, Prolactin, and Cortisol Release in Patients with Anorexia Nervosa." *Journal of Clinical Endocrinology and Metabolism* 91, no. 4 (2006): 1491–1495.

Minuchin, S., B. Rosman, and L. Baker. *Psychosomatic Families: Anorexia Nervosa in Context*. Cambridge: Harvard University Press, 1978.

Nasser, Mervat. *Culture and Weight Consciousness*. London: Routledge, 1997.

National Association of Anorexia Nervosa and Associated Disorders. http://www.anad.org (accessed April 15, 2008).

National Eating Disorders Association. Laxative Abuse and Complications. http://www.nationaleatingdisorders.org (accessed April 21, 2008).

Newspaper Industry. A Brief History of Newspapers. http://www.newspaper-industry.org/history.html (accessed March 2008).

Norris, M.L., K.M. Boydell, L. Pinhas, and D.K. Katzman. "Ana and the Internet: A Review of Pro-Anorexia Websites." *International Journal of Eating Disorders* 39, no. 6 (2006): 443–447.

Paul Poiret. History of Fashion and Costume. http://www.historyoffashion.com/historyofashion/poiret.html (accessed March 2008).

Pearce, J.M.S. "Sir William Withey Gull (1816–1890)." *European Neurology* 55, no. 1 (2006): 53–56.

Pearce, J.M.S. "Richard Morton: Origins of Anorexia Nervosa." *European Neurology* 52, no. 4 (2004): 191–192.

Peters, Lulu Hunt. *Diet and Health with Key to the Calories*. Chicago: The Reilly and Lee Co., 1918.

Pryor, Tamara, and M. Wiederman. "Personality Features and Expressed Concerns of Adolescents with Eating Disorders." *Adolescence Magazine*, June 1998.

Rollin, Lucy. Twentieth Century Teen Culture by the Decades. Westport: Greenwood Press, 1999.

Ruggiero, G., M. Prandin, and M. Mantero. "Eating Disorders across Europe. Eating Disorders in Italy: A Historical Review." *European Eating Disorders Review* 9: 292–300.

Schlenker, J., S. Caron, and W Halteman. "A Feminist Analysis of Seventeen Magazine: Content Analysis from 1945 to 1995." *Sex Roles: A Journal of Research* 38 (1998).

Scholz, Michael, and Eia Asen. "Multiple Family Therapy with Eating Disordered Adolescents: Concepts and Preliminary Results." *European Eating Disorders Review* 9, no. 1 (January 2001): 33–42.

Scholz, Michael, Maud Rix, Katja Scholz, Krassimir Gantchev, and Volker Thomke. "Multiple Family Therapy for Anorexia Nervosa: Concepts, Experiences, and Results." *Journal of Family Therapy* 27, no. 2 (May 2005): 132–141.

Schwartz, M., J. Thomas, K. Bohan, and L. Vartanian. "Intended and Unintended Effects of an Eating Disorder Educational Program: Impact on Presenter Identity." *International Journal of Eating Disorders* 40, no. 2 (2007): 187–192.

"The Self-Starvers." *Time Magazine.* July 28, 1975.

Selvini Palozzoli, Mara. "Anorexia Nervosa: A Syndrome of the Affluent Society." *Transcultural Psychiatric Research Review* 22 (1985): 199–205.

Serdula, M., E. Collins, D. Williamson, and et al. "Weight Control Practices of U.S. Adolescents and Adults." *Annals of Internal Medicine* 119, no. 7 (1993): 667–671.

Shilts, Tom. Research on Males and Eating Disorders. http://www.nationaleatingdisorders.org/p.asp?WebPage_ID=286&Profile_ID=41154 (accessed April 30, 2008).

Shroff, H., et al. "Features Associated with Excessive Exercise in Women with Eating Disorders." *International Journal of Eating Disorders* 39 (2006): 454–461.

Silber, Tomas. "Anorexia Nervosa in Children and Adolescents: Research Evidence Pointing to a Brain-Based Diathesis Supports New Therapeutic Approaches." To Appear in *Pediatric Health, 2009.*

Silber, Tomas. "Anorexia Nervosa among Children and Adolescents." *Advances in Pediatrics* 52 (2005): 49–76.

Silverman, Joseph. "Robert Whytt, 1714–1766, Eighteenth Century Limner of Anorexia Nervosa and Bulimia, an Essay." *International Journal of Eating Disorders* 6, no. 1 (1987): 143–146.

Silverman, Joseph. "Louis-Victor Marcé, 1828: Anorexia Nervosa's Forgotten Man." *Psychological Medicine* 79 (1987): 833–835.

Silverman, Joseph. "Anorexia Nervosa in Seventeenth Century England as Viewed by Physician, Philosopher and Pedagogue." *International Journal of Eating Disorders* 2, no. 4 (1983): 847–853.

Slade, Roger. *The Anorexia Nervosa Reference Book.* London: Harper Collins Publisher Ltd., 1984.

Solomon, Barbara. *In the Company of Educated Women: A History of Women and Higher Education in America.* New Haven: Yale University Press, 1985.

Steffen, K.J., J.L. Roerig, J.E. Mitchell, and S. Uppala. "Emerging Drugs for Eating Disorders Treatment." *Expert Opinion* 11, no. 2 (2006): 315–336.

Striegel-Moore, R., and S. Wonderlich. "Diagnosis and Classification of Eating Disorders: Finding the Way Forward." *International Journal of Eating Disorders* 40 (2007): 21.

Strober, M., R. Freeman, C. Lampert, J. Diamond, and W. Kaye. "Controlled Family Study of Anorexia Nervosa and Bulimia Nervosa: Evidence of Shared Liability and Transmission of Partial Syndromes." *American Journal of Psychiatry* 157, no. 3 (2000): 393–401.

"Teen Age Danger–Dieting until Death." *Port Arthur News.* September 7, 1969.

Tozzi, F., A.W. Bergen, and C.M. Bulik. "Candidate Gene Studies in Eating Disorders." *Psychopharmacology Bulletin* 36, no. 3 (2002): 60–90.

Treasure, J., U. Schmidt, and E. Van Furth. *Handbook of Eating Disorders*. Hoboken: John Wiley & Sons, 2003.

Turner, S., H. Hamilton, M. Jacobs, L. Angood, and D. Dwyer. "The Influence of Fashion Magazines on the Body Image Satisfaction of College Women: An Exploratory Analysis." *Business Network*, Fall 1997.

van Deth, Ron, and Walter Vandereycken. "Food Refusal and Insanity: Sitophobia and Anorexia Nervosa in Victorian Asylums." *International Journal of Eating Disorders* 27, no. 4 (2000): 390–404.

———. *From Fasting Saints to Anorexic Girls*. New York: New York University Press, 1994.

———. "Miraculous Maids? Self-Starving and Fasting Girls." *History Today*, August 1993: 37.

Vandereycken, Walter. "Media Influences and Body Dissatisfaction in Young Women." *Eating Disorders Review* 17, no. 2 (2006): 5.

———. "Organization and Evaluation of an Inpatient Treatment Program for Eating Disorders." *Behavioral Residential Treatment* 3, no. 2 (April 1988): 153–165.

Women's History in America. http://www.wic.org/misc/history.htm (accessed March 2008).

World Health Organization. International Statistical Classification of Diseases and Related Health Problems (ICD-10), 10th Revision. Geneva: World Health Organization, 1992.

Young, Adena. Battling Anorexia: The Story of Karen Carpenter. http://atdpweb.soe.berkeley.edu/quest/Mind&Body/Carpenter.html (accessed March 2008).

YWCA. Beauty at Any Cost. http://www.ywca.com (accessed August 28, 2008).

Zuckerman, Mary Ellen. *A History of Popular Women's Magazines in the United States, 1792–1995*. Westport: Greenwood Press, 1998.

Index

About the Author

STACY BELLER STRYER, M.D. is a graduate of Wellesley College and Yale University School of Medicine. She spent several years working with children and adults with mental illnesses, both in private and public settings. After she completed her pediatric residency at Children's Hospital of Northern California, she joined the Indian Health Service, serving as a staff physician and coordinator of the Kayenta Service Unit's health promotion/disease prevention program. She has consulted for the National Institutes of Health Office of Science Education, Matthews Media Group, Revolution Health, and currently is both a consultant and a regular contributor to the online health Web site, GetbetterHealth, and a board certified pediatrician at Children's First Pediatrics in Rockville, MD